BEHAVIORAL COMPLICATIONS IN ALZHEIMER'S DISEASE

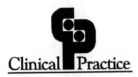

Clinical Practice

Number 31

Judith H. Gold, M.D., F.R.C.P.C.
Series Editor

BEHAVIORAL COMPLICATIONS IN ALZHEIMER'S DISEASE

Edited by

Brian A. Lawlor, M.D., F.R.C.P.I., M.R.C.Psych.

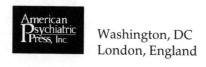

Washington, DC
London, England

Note: The authors have worked to ensure that all information in this book concerning drug dosages, schedules, and routes of administration is accurate as of the time of publication and consistent with standards set by the U.S. Food and Drug Administration and the general medical community. As medical research and practice advance, however, therapeutic standards may change. For this reason and because human and mechanical errors sometimes occur, we recommend that readers follow the advice of a physician who is directly involved in their care or the care of a member of their family.

Copyright © 1995 American Psychiatric Press, Inc.
ALL RIGHTS RESERVED
Manufactured in the United States of America on acid-free paper
First Edition   98 97 96 95   4 3 2 1

American Psychiatric Press, Inc.
1400 K Street, N.W., Washington, DC 20005

Library of Congress Cataloging-in-Publication Data
Behavioral complications in Alzheimer's disease / edited by Brian A.
  Lawlor.
      p.   cm. — (Clinical practice ; no. 31)
    "Based on a symposium held at the 144th Annual Meeting of the
American Psychiatric Association in New Orleans in May 1991"—Pref.
    Includes bibliographical references and index.
    ISBN 0-88048-477-2
    1. Alzheimer's disease—Patients—Mental health—Congresses.
  2. Alzheimer's disease—Complications—Congresses.   I. Lawlor,
  Brian A., 1956- .   II. American Psychiatric Association.   Meeting (144th :
  1991 : New Orleans, La.)   III. Series.
    [DNLM: 1. Alzheimer's Disease—psychology—congresses.
  2. Alzheimer's Disease—complications—congresses.   3. Behavior—
  congresses.   W1 CL767J no. 31 1995]
  RC523.B44   1995
  616.8'31—dc20
  DNLM/DLC
  for Library of Congress   94-38061
                                                                            CIP

British Library Cataloguing in Publication Data
A CIP record is available from the British Library.

Contents

Section I: Phenomenology of Behavioral Disturbance

Section II: Biomedical and Quantitative Aspects of Behavioral Symptoms

Section III: Management Strategies

Section IV: Psychosocial Impact

Contributors

Paul S. Aisen, M.D.
Assistant Professor of Psychiatry, Department of Psychiatry, Mount Sinai School of Medicine of the City University of New York, New York, New York

Stephen M. Aronson, M.D.
Research Fellow, Geriatric Psychiatry Program, University of Michigan Medical School, Ann Arbor, Michigan

Marc Cantillon, M.D.
Medical Staff Fellow, Section on Geriatric Psychiatry, National Institute of Mental Health, Bethesda, Maryland

Lorna S. Carlin, M.D.
Geriatric Psychiatry Research Fellow, Department of Psychiatry, Mount Sinai School of Medicine of the City University of New York, New York, New York

Carl I. Cohen, M.D.
Professor of Psychiatry, Downstate Medical Center, Brooklyn, New York

Christopher C. Colenda III, M.D., M.P.H.
Associate Professor of Psychiatry and Associate in Public Health Sciences, Bowman Gray School of Medicine of Wake Forest University, Winston-Salem, North Carolina

D. P. Devanand, M.D.
Associate Professor of Clinical Psychiatry, Columbia University College of Physicians and Surgeons, and Research Psychiatrist, New York State Psychiatric Institute, New York, New York

Blaine S. Greenwald, M.D.
Associate Professor of Psychiatry, Albert Einstein School of
Medicine of Yeshiva University, Bronx, New York, and
Director, Division of Geriatric Psychiatry, Hillside Hospital,
Long Island Jewish Medical Center, Glen Oaks, New York

Renata Hartung, B.A.
Research Assistant, Department of Psychiatry, State University
of New York, Brooklyn, New York

Brian A. Lawlor, M.D., F.R.C.P.I., M.R.C.Psych.
Consultant in Old Age Psychiatry, St. James's Hospital, and
Senior Lecturer, Department of Psychiatry, University of
Dublin, Trinity College, Dublin, Ireland

John T. Little, M.D.
Senior Staff Fellow, Biological Psychiatry Branch, National
Institute of Mental Health, Bethesda, Maryland

Carol Magai, Ph.D.
Assistant Professor of Psychiatry, State University of New York,
Brooklyn, New York

Alan M. Mellow, M.D., Ph.D.
Director, Geriatric Psychiatry Program and Assistant Professor
of Psychiatry, University of Michigan Medical School, Ann
Arbor, Michigan

Susan E. Molchan, M.D.
Staff Psychiatrist, Section on Geriatric Psychiatry, National
Institute of Mental Health, Bethesda, Maryland

Shirish Patel, M.B.B.S., M.R.C.Psych.
Research Fellow in Psychiatry, Department of Psychiatry,
University of Rochester School of Medicine and Dentistry,
Rochester, New York

Michael Serby, M.D.
Residency Training Director and Associate Professor of
Psychiatry, Department of Psychiatry, Mount Sinai School of
Medicine of the City University of New York, New York, New
York

Trey Sunderland, M.D.
Chief, Section on Geriatric Psychiatry, National Institute of
Mental Health, Bethesda, Maryland

Gregory R. J. Swanwick, M.B., M.R.C.P.I., M.R.C.Psych.
Research Registrar, Mercer's Institute for Research in Ageing,
St. James's Hospital, Dublin, Ireland

Pierre N. Tariot, M.D.
Director, Psychiatry Unit, Monroe Regional Hospital, and
Associate Professor of Psychiatry, University of Rochester
School of Medicine and Dentistry, Rochester, New York

Introduction
to the Clinical Practice Series

O ver the years of its existence the series of monographs entitled *Clinical Insights* gradually became focused on providing current, factual, and theoretical material of interest to the clinician working outside a hospital setting. To reflect this orientation, the name of the Series has been changed to *Clinical Practice*.

The Clinical Practice Series will provide books that give the mental health clinician a practical, clinical approach to a variety of psychiatric problems. These books will provide up-to-date literature reviews and emphasize the most recent treatment methods. Thus, the publications in the Series will interest clinicians working both in psychiatry and in the other mental health professions.

Each year a number of books will be published dealing with all aspects of clinical practice. In addition, from time to time when appropriate, the publications may be revised and updated. Thus, the Series will provide quick access to relevant and important areas of psychiatric practice. Some books in the Series will be authored by a person considered to be an expert in that particular area; others will be edited by such an expert, who will also draw together other knowledgeable authors to produce a comprehensive overview of that topic.

Some of the books in the Clinical Practice Series will have their foundation in presentations at an annual meeting of the American Psychiatric Association. All will contain the most recently available information on the subjects discussed. Theoretical and scientific data will be applied to clinical situations, and case illustrations will be utilized in order to make the material even more relevant for the practitioner. Thus, the Clinical Practice Series should provide educational reading in a compact format especially designed for the mental health clinician–psychiatrist.

Judith H. Gold, M.D., F.R.C.P.C.
Series Editor
Clinical Practice Series

Clinical Practice Series Titles

Successful Psychiatric Practice: Current Dilemmas, Choices, and Solutions (#33)
Edited by Edward K. Silberman, M.D.

Alternatives to Hospitalization for Acute Psychiatric Treatment (#32)
Edited by Richard Warner, M.B., D.P.M.

Behavioral Complications in Alzheimer's Disease (#31)
Edited by Brian A. Lawlor, M.D., F.R.C.P.I., M.R.C.Psych.

Patient Violence and the Clinician (#30)
Edited by Burr S. Eichelman, M.D., Ph.D., and
Anne C. Hartwig, J.D., Ph.D.

Effective Use of Group Therapy in Managed Care (#29)
Edited by K. Roy MacKenzie, M.D., F.R.C.P.C.

Rediscovering Childhood Trauma: Historical Casebook and Clinical Applications (#28)
Edited by Jean M. Goodwin, M.D., M.P.H.

Treatment of Adult Survivors of Incest (#27)
Edited by Patricia L. Paddison, M.D.

Madness and Loss of Motherhood: Sexuality, Reproduction, and Long-Term Mental Illness (#26)
Edited by Roberta J. Apfel, M.D., M.P.H., and
Maryellen H. Handel, Ph.D.

Psychiatric Aspects of Symptom Management in Cancer Patients (#25)
Edited by William Breitbart, M.D., and Jimmie C. Holland, M.D.

Responding to Disaster: A Guide for Mental Health Professionals (#24)
Edited by Linda S. Austin, M.D.

Psychopharmacological Treatment Complications in the Elderly (#23)
Edited by Charles A. Shamoian, M.D., Ph.D.

Anxiety Disorders in Children and Adolescents (#22)
By Syed Arshad Husain, M.D., F.R.C.P.C., F.R.C.Psych., and
Javad Kashani, M.D.

Preface

*U*ntil recently, the primary focus of the pharmacotherapeutics of Alzheimer's disease has been the modification of cognitive impairment. Although the illness is associated with progressive cognitive deterioration, behavioral and psychiatric symptoms are also commonplace and are increasingly being recognized as part of the neurobiology of the disease process. Psychiatric and behavioral disturbances were prominent and integral parts of Alzheimer's first case in 1907, and they still represent one of the more modifiable and potentially treatable aspects of this enigmatic degenerative brain disease.

This book reflects the growing interest in the noncognitive disturbances associated with Alzheimer's disease and is based on a symposium held at the 144th Annual Meeting of the American Psychiatric Association in New Orleans in May 1991. Although there is greater awareness about the impact of behavioral symptoms on patients and caregivers, the phenomenology of these symptoms and the approach to their management are far from standardized. By and large, psychiatrists are unsuccessful in treating many of the behavioral disturbances associated with Alzheimer's disease, and patients with these symptoms consequently require hospitalization and, as a last resort, institutionalization. Interestingly, in spite of the extent of this problem, there is a dearth of controlled studies with pharmacological agents in the treatment of behavioral complications in Alzheimer's disease patients, and the clinician is left somewhat foundering when it comes to dealing with a difficult case.

The aim of the book is to provide clinicians with new information that will guide their clinical management of behaviorally disturbed Alzheimer's disease patients. The recent research on this important topic is reviewed comprehensively, and every attempt is made to relate practical management strategies to emerging research data. Case histories and illustrations are used liberally throughout the book to ground the reader as much as possible in clinical reality.

The impact of behavioral symptoms on the caregiver in terms of burden and stress is considerable. Due consideration is also given to this aspect of the problem, underscoring the fact that in the care of Alzheimer's disease patients, there is also a family or caregiver that may require intervention or help.

This book, and the symposium on which it is based, could not have been possible without the contributions and support of my friends and colleagues who continue to share a special interest in these patients. If this book helps in some small way to dispel the therapeutic nihilism that so often envelops us as we confront Alzheimer's disease patients, the effort and time put into its compilation will have been worthwhile.

Brian A. Lawlor, M.D., F.R.C.P.I., M.R.C.Psych.

Foreword
Behavioral Complications in Alzheimer's Disease

Are behavioral disturbances in Alzheimer's disease complications of the progressive cognitive impairment, or are they really primary manifestations of a devastating brain disease? This question has not been adequately addressed in the scientific literature, as is best exemplified by the discrepancy between the complaints of families about their loved ones and the labeling of symptoms by professionals. For example, although Alzheimer's disease is generally defined by scientists and clinical specialists antemortem as a progressive deterioration of cognitive abilities, families of Alzheimer's disease patients often describe the stages of the illness with behavioral and not cognitive markers. The real-life measures of disease progression are not simply the Mini-Mental State Exam or the Buschke Selective Reminding Task, but rather include the amount of sleeplessness at night, the degree of agitation or psychosis during the day, and the level of depressed mood. The unanswered scientific question is how central these behavioral symptoms are to the heterogeneous biological process we call Alzheimer's disease.

The focus of this book is on the identification, measurement, and treatment of behavioral symptoms in Alzheimer's disease patients. In the section on the phenomenology of behavioral disturbance, there are three chapters in which the authors describe the most common behavioral complications encountered in Alzheimer's disease patients: agitation, psychosis, and depression. Dr. Colenda discusses the description, assessment, and proper diagnosis of agitation in Alzheimer's disease patients. He points out that the symptoms of agitation often represent the final common pathway for many stresses, including a loss of communication skills, psychosis, depression, medical comorbidity, and even iatrogenic factors resulting from medication misjudgments by physicians. And although agitation itself does not represent a separate diagnostic category, its presence should be used as an important warning signal for all clinicians, particularly because agitation often leads to aggressive behavior, which in turn can prematurely precipitate admission to a nursing home.

Depression is perhaps more readily recognized today in Alzheimer's disease patients because of the work over the last 12 years of Burton Reifler and many others (Reifler et al. 1982). Nonetheless, it is generally agreed clinically that depression in these patients is still underdiagnosed and undertreated. Considering that the efficacy of antidepressant treatments in this group is similar to that in all other elderly populations, this potential oversight has unfortunate implications. Dr. Greenwald, in his thoughtful chapter, addresses these and many more issues, including the all-important psychosocial context of the Alzheimer's disease patient. Although having Alzheimer's disease may in itself be depressing, it should never be used as an excuse for not aggressively evaluating and treating a potentially reversible aspect of the illness. Dr. Molchan and her colleagues, in their chapter on psychotic symptoms in Alzheimer's disease, next address the diverse phenomenology of psychosis in the illness. Although clusters of common symptoms as well as idiosyncratic psychotic manifestations have now been identified in the literature, there is still a great need for further cross-sectional and longitudinal studies, from both a biological and a clinical perspective. Dr. Molchan makes the very important point that these studies may help illuminate the underlying biology of other psychotic syndromes in addition to Alzheimer's disease. Furthermore, these insights might lead to treatment advances across a spectrum of behavioral disorders, including Alzheimer's disease.

In the section on biomedical and quantitative aspects, there are three chapters summarizing a great deal of information. First, Dr. Aisen reviews the all-important need for careful coordination between physicians in the treatment of patients with dementia. That need is obvious at the time of initial diagnosis, but the concept of coordinated care is often overlooked at later times when "complications" arise. Dr. Little then reviews the use of behavioral rating scales in Alzheimer's disease. Although earlier research in this area suffered from a paucity of reliable rating instruments, it should be clear after reading this chapter that such a drought no longer exists. Rather, the problem is now probably the opposite, and the field needs to establish consistent standards for behavioral measurement across studies. From a biological perspective, Dr. Lawlor next examines the pathological changes commonly reported in Alzheimer's disease studies. The implicit hope is that focusing on neurotransmitter abnormalities outside the well-documented cholinergic changes can expand the potential treatment armamentarium. As an added benefit, clinicopathological similarities between dementia and other psychiatric disorders may lead to new insights regarding those illnesses as well.

In the third section of the book, on management strategies, appears a most complete collection of guidelines for the treatment of behavioral manifestations of Alzheimer's disease. Dr. Devanand starts the section with a review of neuroleptic use. While pointing out that adequate rigorous research is not yet available to address many important therapeutic questions, he provides a practical guide to the clinical use of neuroleptics in patients with dementia. Similarly, Drs. Patel and Tariot point out that the use of benzodiazepines is not well studied in Alzheimer's disease. In fact, they suggest that careful trials of discontinuing long-term benzodiazepine therapy may be of significant benefit to patients, because so many have been receiving long-term benzodiazepines for unclear reasons. Dr. Serby's chapter urges caution in the treatment of depression in dementia. Although antidepressants, electroconvulsive therapy, and other nonmedication approaches such as psychotherapy may be helpful in some cases, careful attention to side effects must be exercised. Dr. Serby emphasizes that family interventions may be the most therapeutic approach available. Dr. Swanwick continues this emphasis by focusing on nonpharmacological approaches to behavioral disturbances. However, he is quick to point out that there is surprisingly little research to support one medical or nonmedical intervention over another. Given the obvious economic advantages of less-restrictive management options, this area needs much further study. Because there is a lack of clear-cut efficacy in the standard pharmacological treatments, Drs. Mellow and Aronson's review of new pharmacological approaches for behavioral management in Alzheimer's disease is extremely important. Although this research is still relatively underdeveloped, the breadth of innovative approaches (from anticonvulsants to beta-blockers) is impressive and worthy of careful attention in upcoming years.

In the fourth and final section of the book are two chapters that bring the focus back to the all-important psychosocial implications of behavioral symptoms in Alzheimer's disease: 1) caregiver burden and 2) disposition dilemmas. Dr. Magai and colleagues discuss the rapidly expanding but generally inconclusive data on caregiver strain and its relationship to severity of dementia and behavioral complications. Correctly, they point out the need to focus future research on the social impact, both economic and personal, of continued home management of Alzheimer's disease patients. Drs. Carlin and Lawlor then draw the connection between behavioral disturbances in Alzheimer's disease and institutional support. They emphasize that long-term care is not synonymous with nursing home placement, but that there is a diverse spectrum of possibilities that need to be examined carefully for therapeutic usefulness and socioeconomic impact.

In summary, the emphasis of this book is on the phenomenology of behavioral symptoms in Alzheimer's disease and related treatment issues. From that perspective, it is clearly an optimistic endeavor that should be of great value to interested clinicians and researchers. Perhaps more important, however, in this book the stage is set for further investigations in each of the areas outlined. Although very few conclusive research data are available at this time, the book documents a growing interest in future studies and the necessary methodological infrastructure for them. We cannot yet answer the question posed at the beginning of this introduction—whether behavioral symptoms represent a primary or secondary manifestation of Alzheimer's disease pathology—but we can effectively pursue related questions. For instance, why is it that a significant percentage of late-onset depressive patients go on to develop dementia (Kral 1983; Reding et al. 1985)? Could it be that behavioral symptoms might even be the initial diagnostic markers in some cases of Alzheimer's disease? Are there different prognostic or therapeutic implications for Alzheimer's disease patients with behavioral complications and those without them? These are the research questions of the near future.

In the meantime, some partially effective treatments for the behavioral manifestations of Alzheimer's disease are available, and numerous others are under study. This state of affairs reflects major progress during the last 10 years, and many of the decade's advances are chronicled in this book.

Trey Sunderland, M.D.

References

Kral VA: The relationship between senile dementia (Alzheimer type) and depression. Can J Psychiatry 28:304–306, 1983

Reding M, Haycox J, Blass J: Depression in patients referred to a dementia clinic: a three-year prospective study. Arch Neurol 42:894–896, 1985

Reifler BV, Larson E, Hanley R: Coexistence of cognitive impairment and depression in geriatric outpatients. Am J Psychiatry 139:623–626, 1982

Section I

Phenomenology of Behavioral Disturbance

CHAPTER 1

Agitation:
A Conceptual Overview

Christopher C. Colenda III, M.D., M.P.H.

*A*gitated patients with dementia behave in a manner that may place themselves and others in danger (Maletta 1990), contribute to a great deal of distress and burden for caregivers (Chenoweth and Spencer 1986; Everitt et al. 1991; Sanford 1975), and severely disrupt family, social, and institutional networks. Agitated behaviors are frequent reasons for acute hospitalization and long-term institutional placement (Moak 1990). From a clinical point of view, the development of agitated behavior is the primary reason why health care professionals are asked to intervene with behavioral or pharmacological treatments. Although interventions are obviously needed for these patients, the amount of available research that establishes the efficacy of different treatments is relatively small, leading many physicians to feel a degree of therapeutic nihilism when it comes to dealing with these patients.

This work is supported in part by the Geriatric Mental Health Academic Award of the National Institute of Mental Health (K07-MH00787).

Defining *Agitation* in Alzheimer's Disease

Although the term *agitated* is frequently used to describe the behavior of a patient with Alzheimer's disease, an imprecise definition has led to a confusing picture of exactly what behaviors should and should not be considered agitated. In turn, ambiguity over what should be viewed as agitation can contribute to uncertain clinical judgments about how best to treat these behaviors. For example, clinicians will often be asked to "do something" for a wandering patient with dementia who becomes physically "agitated" when caregivers try to curb the patient's behavior. Should the clinician primarily address the patient's wandering, address the interventions the caregiver used that resulted in the escalation of violence, or make recommendations for curbing the physical aggression itself? Obviously, all three interacting behavioral components need to be addressed. But often, busy clinicians do not have the time to reconstruct the events that led to the phone call asking for urgent therapeutic action.

Agitated behaviors may also represent signs and symptoms of undetected comorbid psychiatric illness, such as depression, psychosis, or delirium. In these instances the manifest symptoms of agitation are the behavioral translation of psychic anxiety, hallucinations, perceptual disturbances, delusions, and worsening cognitive function. Prompt recognition and treatment of the underlying psychiatric symptoms may greatly diminish the patient's propensity to act out aggressively.

An operational definition of agitation has been proposed and developed by Cohen-Mansfield and colleagues on the basis of a series of empirical studies conducted with agitated nursing home residents. Although these studies included subjects who did not necessarily have dementia, the definition of agitation was developed from empirical evidence of patient behavior. This body of research also strengthens the perspective that agitated behaviors are not monolithic, but can be factored into separate categories, which in turn may improve diagnostic and treatment specificity. Cohen-Mansfield and Billig (1986) postulated three requirements for an operational definition of agitation:

1) The definition should be an operational one, based on observable behavior; 2) "agitation" should not include behaviors which are known to occur generally due to factors other than agitation. This requirement excludes sleep disturbances or falls from the definition of agitation per se; 3) "agitation" excludes behaviors which can be explained otherwise; i.e., a purposeful walk or an occasional walk of a confused elderly person who loses his way. ... Agitation is ... defined as inappropriate verbal, vocal, or motor activity that is not explained by needs or confusion, per se. It includes behaviors such as aimless wandering, pacing, cursing, screaming, biting, and fighting. (p. 771)

Inappropriate is further characterized as abusive, aggressive, or socially inappropriate behaviors. Of the 29 symptoms of agitation listed in the Cohen-Mansfield Agitation Inventory (CMAI) (Cohen-Mansfield et al. 1989), factor analysis suggests that agitated behaviors can be organized into a three-factor model: aggressive behavior (including physical and verbal), physically nonaggressive behavior (such as pacing, restlessness, wandering), and verbally agitated behaviors (such as screaming, repeated requests for attention). The three-factor model distinguishes agitation from psychiatric symptoms manifested by Alzheimer's disease patients, such as anxiety, depression, hallucinations, and delusions. Although psychiatric symptoms may make the Alzheimer's disease patient vulnerable to agitation, they do not always accompany agitation (Colenda 1991; Maletta 1990).

Developing a Conceptual Framework for Agitation in Alzheimer's Disease

Clearly, agitated behaviors and other psychiatric symptoms rarely occur as individual or isolated events. More commonly, they cluster together (Baker et al. 1991; Cohen-Mansfield et al. 1989). For example, Baker's group (1991) found that 69 (or 57%) of 122 Alzheimer's disease patients demonstrated mixed psychiatric and behavioral symptoms. Cohen-Mansfield's work has also demonstrated that symptoms of agitation cluster in the following schemes: hitting with cursing and pushing; kicking with hitting, pushing, and scratching; inappropriate dressing with pacing; handling things inappropriately; and general restlessness (Cohen-Mansfield 1986; Cohen-Mansfield and Billig 1986). Because behaviors tend to cluster, clinicians may have difficulty discriminating whether the symptoms can be treated with a single intervention, such as a medication, or whether a more complex treatment approach is needed. For example, if a patient is verbally abusive to a caregiver and was also found to be paranoid, prescribing a neuroleptic medication might diminish the agitated verbal behavior. On the other hand, verbally intrusive outbursts that are secondary to attention-seeking behavior may not be responsive to medications alone, but may require a more coordinated treatment effort designed to reward the patient for not exhibiting attention-seeking behavior.

Another feature of agitation different from the core cognitive disturbance is its fluctuating nature. In contrast to memory loss, which is inexorably progressive, agitated behaviors are usually episodic and emergent and may often occur in response to environmental and social cues. For example, research has shown that physical agitation may increase when caregivers try to get Alzheimer's disease patients to maintain self-care or engage in other routine activities of daily living (Cohen-Mansfield and Billig 1986; Cohen-Mansfield et al. 1989; Colenda and Hamer 1991). But because agitation can be spontaneous and at times seemingly random and without identifiable causes (Colenda and Hamer 1991), clinicians may also have the burden of formulating treatment plans without a clear sense of the events that preceded the aggressive outburst. In this situation they are required to react fast and to choose treatments that can bring the situation quickly under control. The urgency of the clinical situation, clinical uncertainty about the efficacy of behavioral interventions as well as inexperience in how to effectively employ them, and the possibility that comorbid medical and psychiatric conditions may be contributing to the current crisis may result in physicians' over-reliance on psychotropic medication as the main intervention strategy (Colenda 1991; Everitt et al. 1991).

For example, a 78-year-old Alzheimer's disease patient living in a nursing home became acutely agitated, emotionally labile, and restless over the course of several days. Her local physician, who knew the patient well, prescribed lorazepam over the phone. This helped initially, but after 3 days of increasingly agitated behavior, she was seen in the office. There it was discovered that she had an *Escherichia coli* urinary tract infection. Antibiotic treatment of the infection successfully treated her agitation.

Other factors have been shown to influence agitation in Alzheimer's disease patients. Clinical evidence suggests that noncognitive agitated behaviors are linked to the patient's level of the cognitive impairment—for example, the more cognitively impaired the patient, the more likely it is that the patient will evidence agitated behavior (Cooper et al. 1990; Teri et al. 1988). Others have found that the early development of psychotic symptoms correlates with a more rapid decline in cognitive abilities (Drevets and Rubin 1989). Although this relationship is potentially useful as prognostic information, caution about its generalizability is recommended, because the number of psychotic patients used to make the comparison was small. The risk of agitation has also been shown to be higher for male dementia patients (Cariaga et al. 1991; Cooper et al. 1990). Additionally, specific behaviors, such as screaming and vocal outbursts, are strongly correlated with increased functional impairment, depressed affect, and social networks of poor quality (Cariaga et al. 1991; Cohen-Mansfield and Marx 1988; Cohen-Mansfield et al. 1990).

Thus, the available evidence is convincing that the development and perpetuation of agitated behavior in Alzheimer's disease patients is best conceptualized as a function of the interactive effects of patient characteristics, cognitive functioning, social and environmental networks, and the unrelenting progression of the illness.

Prevalence Rates of Agitated Behaviors and Selected Psychiatric Symptoms in Alzheimer's Disease

The importance of having accurate prevalence estimates of agitated behaviors and psychiatric symptoms in patients with Alzheimer's disease rests on the fundamental principle of medical decision making. That is, accurate baseline prevalence information has been shown to be a critical component in making appropriate medical decisions (Baron et al. 1988; Christensen-Szalanski and Beach 1982; Einhorn and Hogarth 1978; Gruppen et al. 1991; Hershey and Baron 1987). When accurate estimates of behavioral and psychiatric symptoms in dementia patients are not available, physicians may experience increasing uncertainty about how to manage these patients, fail to detect treatable symptoms, have narrower treatment choices, and be at greater risk of misapplying treatments, particularly with regard to pharmacological interventions.

Unfortunately, establishing accurate estimates of prevalence rates for psychiatric and behavioral problems in Alzheimer's disease patients has been plagued by a number of problems, discussed here in four general categories.

First, the prevalence of psychiatric and behavioral symptoms appears to depend on how cognitively impaired patients are— for example, patients with advanced cognitive impairment have more symptoms than those who are less impaired (Cooper et al. 1990; Drevets and Rubin 1989; Teri et al. 1988).

Second, many reports use relatively small patient samples drawn from clinical settings in which patients are more likely to exhibit behavioral and psychiatric symptoms, such as nursing homes and mental institutions. Hence, reported prevalence rates may actually overestimate the scope of these symptoms when all Alzheimer's disease patients are considered. For example, because aggressive behaviors have been found to be major risk factors for institutionalization (Burns et al. 1990; Colenda and Hamer 1991; Moak 1990), it is not surprising that institutionalized patients have higher rates of psychiatric and behavioral symptoms. A recent report by Eisdorfer and colleagues (1992) has significantly advanced our knowledge about the prevalence of specific behaviors and psychiatric symptoms in community-dwelling Alzheimer's disease patients. Although the report primarily focused on examining the validity of the Global Deterioration Scale (GDS) (Reisberg et al. 1988), the authors examined the prevalence of specific symptoms in a large sample of patients stratified by an estimate of disease severity. The results revealed that behavioral and psychiatric symptoms are quite prevalent and do not necessarily occur late in the disease course.

Third, behavioral and psychiatric symptoms are not defined or listed in clinical and research reports in a consistent manner. For example, some authors treat delusions and hallucinations as separate clinical symptoms (Ballinger et al. 1982; Eisdorfer et al. 1992; Reisberg et al. 1987), whereas others collapse the two symptoms into a single category (Cooper 1990; Swearer et al. 1988). Although separating these symptoms may have some utility from a research perspective, it may be less important clinically, because their presence is good evidence for psychotic thinking— essentially what clinicians should be trying to detect. Identifying evidence of psychotic thinking, in the form of hallucinations and delusions, may better define and focus treatment options.

However, merely finding these symptoms in Alzheimer's disease patients may not be enough, especially for the inexperienced clinician. For example, delusions and hallucinations may represent symptoms of comorbid delirium, medication intoxication, or severe depression. Hence, treating these underlying conditions may represent better approaches to patient care than merely administering neuroleptic medications. Accordingly, as clinicians attempt to better describe psychiatric and behavioral symptoms in their patients, differential diagnoses and treatment options may increase. Expanding our knowledge of the potential sources of agitation and psychiatric symptoms in these patients may ironically lead to an increase in clinicians' initial uncertainty about treatment options (Christensen-Szalanski and Beach 1982; Hershey and Baron 1987). However, as clinicians expand their knowledge base, treatments may become more diverse and focused, ultimately leading to better patient care.

Fourth, until Cohen-Mansfield's work, an empirically derived classification of agitation has not been available. Without a uniform definition, reported prevalence rates are difficult to interpret with any degree of confidence. For example, some investigators use *agitation* or *aggression* to refer to physical aggression alone (Baker et al. 1991; Eisdorfer et al. 1992; Reisberg et al. 1987). Cohen-Mansfield, however, separates physical from vocal agitated behaviors (Cohen-Mansfield 1986; Cohen-Mansfield et al. 1989), which expands the scope of the definition but also raises conceptual questions about whether vocal and physical agitation should be given similar clinical weight in terms of severity estimate and treatment strategy.

These caveats notwithstanding, Tables 1–1 and 1–2 summarize behavioral and psychiatric prevalence rates gathered from research reports (Ballinger et al. 1982; Burns et al. 1990; Cohen-Mansfield 1986; Eisdorfer et al. 1992; Reifler et al. 1982; Reisberg et al. 1987; Swearer et al. 1988; Teri et al. 1988). A number of criteria were used to decide which reports were included in the final tabulation.

First, articles had to report the size of the patient sample and the actual number of patients demonstrating the particular symptom. Second, behavioral and psychiatric symptoms had to be individually listed in the articles. Because not all authors listed symptoms the same way, however, several symptoms were merged into single categories for this chapter, for example, physical aggression/agitation, verbal aggression/threats, sleep disturbances, apathy/withdrawal, and all mood disturbances and paranoia/suspiciousness. Third, because the frequencies of some behaviors were so small (such as fearfulness and binge eating), they were excluded from the final tabulation. And last, because the primary goal was generating estimated mean prevalence rates with standard deviations for selected symptoms, symptom categories were included only if data from three separate original reports could be reliably documented.

Table 1–1 presents prevalence information for agitated and disruptive behaviors from eight clinical studies. Verbal aggression/threats (54%) and physical aggression/agitation (42%) constitute the two most frequent agitated behaviors reported in Alzheimer's disease patients. The high mean prevalence rates for both behaviors clearly reinforce the clinical magnitude of these problems for caregivers and clinicians. Other behaviors, however, are also quite prevalent. Sleep disturbances (38%), restlessness (38%), and wandering (30%) constitute additional behavioral burdens of some magnitude. Table 1–2 prevalence rates demonstrate that delusions (50%), hallucinations (24%), and paranoia/suspiciousness (30%) constitute major psychiatric symptoms that cause still more disability for Alzheimer's disease patients. Because psychotic symptoms further compromise a de-

Table 1–1. Prevalence of selected agitated and disruptive behaviors among dementia patients, summarized from eight recent clinical studies

	Size of patient sample	Physical aggression/ agitation		Verbal aggression/ threats		Rest- lessness		Wandering		Sleep distur- bances		Apathy/ with- drawal	
		n	%	n	%	n	%	n	%	n	%	n	%
Ballinger et al. 1982	100	54	54	67	67	–	–	–	–	70	70	–	–
Cohen-Mansfield 1986[a]	66	34	52	43	65	22	33	35	53	–	–	–	–
Reisberg et al. 1987	33	26	79	11	33	12	36	1	3	14	42	1	3
Swearer et al. 1988	126	27	21	64	51	–	–	–	–	55	45	–	–
Teri et al. 1988	127	30	24	–	–	57	45	33	26	–	–	–	–
Burns et al. 1990	178	35	20	–	–	–	–	33	19	–	–	71	41
Cooper et al. 1990	680	365	53	–	–	–	–	180	26	124	18	295	43
Eisdorfer et al. 1992	324	106	33	–	–	–	–	–	–	54	17	70	22
Mean prevalence			42.0 ± 20.9		54.0 ± 15.7		38.0 ± 6.2		29.6 ± 13.4		38.4 ± 22.0		27.3 ± 18.7

Note. Empty cells represent parameters not measured in that study.
[a] Nursing home study (physical aggression included hitting, kicking, and biting).

Table 1–2.   Prevalence of selected psychiatric symptoms among dementia patients summarized from eight recent clinical studies

	Size of patient sample	Mood disturbances (depression, tearful episodes)		Emotional lability		Delusions		Hallucinations		Paranoia/suspiciousness	
		n	%	n	%	n	%	n	%	n	%
Eisdorfer et al. 1992	324	98	30	24	7	39	12	41	13	39	12
Teri et al. 1988	127	—	—	—	—	—	—	27	21	30	24
Burns et al. 1990	178	—	—	—	—	—	—	—	—	—	—
Reisberg et al. 1987[a]	33	8	24	1	3	34	100	8	24	14	42
Swearer et al. 1988[b]	126	—	—	—	—	—	—	28	22	40	32
Cooper et al. 1990[b]	680	201	29	—	—	—	—	213	31	—	—
Ballinger et al. 1982	100	42	42	14	14	38	38	34	34	39	39
Reifler et al. 1982	85	17	20	—	—	—	—	—	—	—	—
Mean prevalence			29.0 ± 8.3		8.0 ± 5.6		50.0 ± 45.2		24.2 ± 7.5		29.8 ± 12.1

Note.   Empty cells represent parameters not measured in that study.
[a]Combined all types of delusions.
[b]Hallucinations and delusions are reported as a single category in the original article.
[c]Final sample size is based on evaluation of the author's raw data.

mentia patient's ability to make rational judgments, it is easy to understand how the high prevalence of these symptoms contributes to patients' vulnerability to the development of agitation. Mood disturbances, primarily reported as depression, were found in 29% of patients in studies reported. It is unclear, however, to what extent symptoms of apathy and withdrawal (27%) represent behavioral proxies for depression in these patients.

The prevalence rates summarized in Tables 1–1 and 1–2 do not provide much insight into the relationships among agitated behaviors, psychiatric symptoms, and other social or environmental cues. Baker and colleagues (1991) reported that 57% of her patient population demonstrated mixed psychiatric symptoms. Symptoms tended to cluster in the following manner: depression occurred with confusion, agitation, and anxiety in 33.9% of patients; agitation accompanied belligerence, fighting, and confusion in 23.7% of patients; and wandering accompanied restlessness, confusion, and anxiety in 18.6% of patients. Deutsch and Rovner (1991) report that Alzheimer's disease patients who were more physically violent were more dependent on caregivers for activities of daily living (ADL), such as washing, oral hygiene, dressing, and toilet needs. Correspondingly, staff-patient interaction was the most frequently identified precipitant for physical aggression in state hospital dementia patients (Colenda and Hamer 1991).

Sleep disturbances have also been strongly correlated with behavioral disturbances during the day, such as wandering or agitation (Rebok et al. 1991). *Sundowning* (the increased prevalence of psychiatric and behavioral symptoms in the early evening) has been linked to changes in sleep patterns (partial arousal from rapid eye movement sleep, sleep apnea, and phase shifting) as well as to sensory deprivation, loneliness, and diminished social and physical time cues (e.g., zeitgebers) (Reynolds 1991). Hence, sundowning may represent an additional behavioral disorder caused partially by sleep disturbances and disrupted circadian rhythms.

Interestingly, agitation and other psychiatric symptoms are not necessarily reserved for the later stages of Alzheimer's disease. Eisdorfer and colleagues (1992) showed that symptoms occur earlier in the disease course than predicted by the Global

Deterioration Scale (GDS) (Reisberg et al. 1988). Specifically, more than 50% of patients had evidence of psychiatric pathology by the time they reached GDS level 2. At GDS level 4, 40% of the patients were agitated; 17% demonstrated delusions; 15% demonstrated hallucinations; 20% were paranoid; and 26% were depressed. In addition, significant increases in the rates of psychiatric symptoms occurred between GDS levels 3 and 4, which is earlier in the illness course than was predicted by the scale. The work of Eisdorfer and colleagues highlights the difficulty of using a single instrument to fully describe the cognitive, functional, and behavioral decline found in Alzheimer's disease patients. They also noted that

> The use of the Global Deterioration Scale as a global staging instrument carries with it the subtle hazard that because the scaled score provides information in a quasi-mathematical form, it can appear to convey more information about the patient's condition than it actually does. (p. 194)

In summary, the available evidence suggests that verbal outbursts, physical aggression, agitation, and wandering are major behavioral problems in Alzheimer's disease patients. Other symptoms such as sleep disturbances, hallucinations, delusions, and paranoia are almost as prevalent, and they probably make patients more vulnerable to agitation. Because correctly identifying psychiatric symptoms may improve the success of pharmacological treatments (Colenda 1991; Maletta 1990), it is important for clinicians to identify them where possible. The clinician is also advised to look for co-occurring medical illnesses that may present with atypical symptoms such as agitation. Finally, evidence suggests that the risk of psychiatric and behavioral symptoms may occur early in the patient's illness and is not necessarily a function of increasing severity of dementia and progression of the disease.

Conclusions

Systematic research confirms that agitated behaviors tend to cluster into three main patterns: physically aggressive behavior, non-physically aggressive behavior, and verbal aggression. It is important for clinicians to look for specific medical and psychiatric symptoms or illnesses that may co-occur in Alzheimer's disease patients and thus predispose them to an increased risk of agitation. Prevalence rates from multiple research reports show that physical and vocal aggression, sleep disturbances, and restlessness are the most prominent behavioral symptoms and that delusions, hallucinations, and paranoia are the most frequent psychiatric symptoms. These frequent noncognitive disturbances in Alzheimer's disease patients contribute to the clinical picture of agitated behavior in these patients but obviously suggest different treatment interventions.

The accurate detection of symptoms and their underlying cause is critical to improving treatment specificity. In this regard, an appreciation of the interaction of environment, physical illness, disease severity, and psychiatric symptomatology in the expression of agitation in an individual patient is key to developing a therapeutic framework for the management of these disturbed behaviors.

References

Baker FM, Kokmen E, Chandra V, et al: Psychiatric symptoms in cases of clinically diagnosed Alzheimer's disease. J Geriatr Psychiatry Neurol 4:71–78, 1991

Ballinger BR, Reid AH, Heather BB: Cluster analysis of symptoms in elderly demented patients. Br J Psychiatry 140:257–262, 1982

Baron J, Beattie J, Hershey JC: Heuristics and biases in diagnostic reasoning, II: congruence, information, and uncertainty. Organizational Behavior and Human Decision Processes 42:88–110, 1988

Burns A, Jacoby R, Levy R: Psychiatric phenomena in Alzheimer's disease, IV: disorders of behavior. Br J Psychiatry 157:86–94, 1990

Cariaga J, Burgio L, Flynn W, Martin D: A controlled study of disruptive vocalizations among geriatric residents in nursing homes. J Am Geriatr Soc 39:501–507, 1991

Chenoweth B, Spencer B: Dementia: the experience of family caregivers. Gerontologist 26:267–272, 1986

Christensen-Szalanski JJJ, Beach LR: Experience and the base-rate fallacy. Organizational Behavior and Human Performance 29:270–279, 1982

Cohen-Mansfield J: Agitated behaviors in the elderly: preliminary results in the cognitively deteriorated. J Am Geriatr Soc 34:722–727, 1986

Cohen-Mansfield J, Billig N: Agitated behaviors in the elderly, I: a conceptual review. J Am Geriatr Soc 34:711–721, 1986

Cohen-Mansfield J, Marx MS: Relationship between depression and agitation in nursing home residents. Comprehensive Gerontology 2:141–146, 1988

Cohen-Mansfield J, Marx MS, Rosenthal AS: A description of agitation in a nursing home. J Gerontol 44(3):M77–84, 1989

Cohen-Mansfield J, Werner P, Marx MS: Screaming in nursing home residents. J Am Geriatr Soc 38:785–792, 1990

Colenda CC: Drug treatment of behavior problems in elderly patients with dementia, I. Drug Therapy 21:15–20, 1991

Colenda CC, Hamer RM: Antecedents and interventions for aggressive behavior of patients at a geropsychiatric state hospital. Hosp Community Psychiatry 42:287–293, 1991

Cooper JK, Mungas D, Weiler PG: Relation of cognitive status and abnormal behaviors in Alzheimer's disease. J Am Geriatr Soc 38:867–870, 1990

Deutsch LH, Rovner BW: Agitation and the other noncognitive abnormalities in Alzheimer's disease. Psychiatr Clin North Am 14:341–351, 1991

Drevets WC, Rubin EH: Psychotic symptoms and the longitudinal course of senile dementia of the Alzheimer's type. Biol Psychiatry 25:39–48, 1989

Einhorn HJ, Hogarth RM: Confidence in judgment: persistence of the illusion of validity. Psychol Rev 85:395–416, 1978

Eisdorfer C, Cohen D, Paveza GJ, et al: An empirical evaluation of the Global Deterioration Scale for staging Alzheimer's disease. Am J Psychiatry 149:190–194, 1992

Everitt DE, Fields DR, Soumerai SB, et al: Resident behavior and staff distress in the nursing home. J Am Geriatr Soc 39:792–798, 1991

Gruppen LD, Wolf FM, Billi JE: Information gathering and integration as sources of error in diagnostic decision making. Med Decis Making 11:233–239, 1991

Hershey JC, Baron J: Clinical reasoning and cognitive processes. Med Decis Making 7:203–211, 1987

Maletta GJ: Pharmacologic treatment and management of the aggressive dementia patient. Psychiatric Annals 20:446–455, 1990

Moak GS: Characteristics of demented and nondemented geriatric admissions to a state hospital. Hosp Community Psychiatry 41:799–801, 1990

Rebok GW, Rovner BW, Folstein MF: Sleep disturbance in Alzheimer's disease: relationship to behavioral problems. Aging 3:193–196, 1991

Reifler BV, Larson E, Hanley R: Coexistence of cognitive impairment and depression in geriatric outpatients. Am J Psychiatry 139:623–626, 1982

Reisberg B, Borenstein J, Salob SP, et al: Behavioral symptoms in Alzheimer's disease: phenomenology and treatment. J Clin Psychiatry 48 (suppl 5):9–15, 1987

Reisberg B, Ferris S, Deleon MJ, et al: Global Deterioration Scale (GDS). Psychopharmacol Bull 24:661–663, 1988

Reynolds CF: Sleep disorders, in Comprehensive Review of Geriatric Psychiatry. Edited by Sadavoy J, Lazarus LW, Jarvik LF. Washington, DC, American Psychiatric Press, 1991, pp 403–418

Sanford JRA: Tolerance of debility in elderly dependents by supporters at home: its significance for hospital practice. BMJ 3:471–473, 1975

Swearer JM, Drachman DA, O'Donnell BF, et al: Troublesome and disruptive behaviors in dementia: relationship to diagnosis and disease severity. J Am Geriatr Soc 36:784–790, 1988

Teri L, Larson EB, Reifler BV: Behavioral disturbance in dementia of the Alzheimer's type. J Am Geriatr Soc 36:1–6, 1988

CHAPTER 2

Depression in Alzheimer's Disease and Related Dementias

Blaine S. Greenwald, M.D.

A considerable body of clinical and scientific work has evolved over the last 10–15 years recognizing that serious and treatable depression may develop in patients with Alzheimer's disease and related dementias. My aim in this chapter is to synthesize this extensive literature. I review clinically relevant historical, epidemiological, pathophysiological, and diagnostic concepts regarding depression complicating preexisting dementia and follow with illustrative case vignettes.

Historical Perspective

That depression may complicate preexisting Alzheimer's disease and related dementias has long been recognized. Classical psychiatric phenomenologists either alluded to or explicitly addressed the phenomenon of affective symptomatology complicating dementia. For example, at the turn of the century, Emil Kraepelin (1904), in discussing senile dementia, described apparent mood-congruent depressive delusions:

Delusions are mostly of a persecutory character; the patients believe they are being neglected, little things are done to annoy them, and finally they are deprived of property. (p. 276)

Kraepelin further comments on emotionality in dementia:

In emotional attitude, there is a variation between elation and depression. [Patients] are irritable, peevish, and discontented. The states of the emotional attitude are both superficial and transitory; extreme and tearful sympathy or silly happiness may be aroused on the slightest pretext. (p. 276)

Eugen Bleuler (1924), in writing about "senile dementia" (probably analogous to today's primary degenerative dementia of the Alzheimer's type, senile onset), noted:

Accessory symptoms can change the picture and often make institutional care necessary. Torpidity can increase to stupor. The mild affective displacements which are frequent in old age can rise to melancholic and manic conditions, of which the first are very frequent ("senile melancholia"), the second rare. The depression is frequently accompanied by anxiety. In such affective conditions, delusions are . . . formed. In depressive delusional forms the delusion of poverty usually recedes before the horribly developed delusion of sin and hypochondriasis. Very often these affective delusions are mingled with delusions of suspicion, self-reference, and of persecution. (pp. 289–290)

Writing about "arteriosclerotic insanity" (presumably analogous to today's term *multi-infarct dementia*), Bleuler continued (edited for brevity):

Undoubtedly there exists a primary tendency to depression and to an anxious conception of experiences. . . . initiative weakens, it becomes difficult to rouse themselves to action . . . affectivity becomes more labile. . . . the patient's interest becomes narrowed and the tendency to depression inhibits somewhat the emotional fluctuations. . . . there is a tendency to real melancholia. Patients become less courageous, they are timid, conceive everything as painful, and form depressive delusions, especially . . . of a hypochondriacal type. (pp. 280–281)

Several ideas of conceptual, diagnostic, and categorical relevance are embedded in these historical excerpts: 1) depression in dementia may occur frequently; 2) depression may exist both as a symptom and as a syndrome in dementia patients; 3) depression may be transient or lasting; 4) affective delusions (e.g., of impoverishment, sin, disease) may suggest depression; 5) in dementia patients, depression may be associated with different presentations, for example, anxiety or apathy; 6) differences may exist between depression in Alzheimer's dementia and in multi-infarct dementia; and 7) depression may complicate and confound the clinical picture of dementia so that institutionalization is hastened, possibly prematurely.

Later, Sir Martin Roth (1955) framed an important nosological distinction by incisively identifying two types of depression in dementia (edited for brevity):

> There were (dementia) cases which had shown at some stage of the illness a *sustained depressive-symptom complex.* . . . There is, however, another type of affective change associated with the organic psychoses (dementias) of old age. . . . The mood change is short-lived and shallow. . . . depressive ideas are fragmentary and transient. . . . This group of cases seems, therefore, to deserve separate consideration from conditions in which a sustained depressive symptom-complex is associated with arteriosclerotic or senile disease. . . . what interpretation is placed upon the incidence of affective symptoms in the senile and arteriosclerotic cases must depend on whether a distinction is maintained between ill-sustained, atypical depressive symptoms and a depressive symptom-complex. (pp. 294–295, 298)

With this in mind, I focus in this chapter on the diagnosis and identification of a *syndrome* of major depression (Roth's *sustained depressive symptom-complex)* complicating preexisting dementia. A growing body of published clinical experience suggests that a major depressive episode complicating dementia is responsive to somatic antidepressant treatment (drugs and electroconvulsive therapy [ECT]) (Cole et al. 1983; Devanand and Nelson 1985; Greenwald et al. 1989a; Haupt 1991; Nelson and Rosenberg 1991; Price and McAllister 1989; Reifler et al. 1989; Reynolds et al. 1988; Snow and Wells 1981). Hence the identification of a major depressive syndrome in a patient with dementia should provoke an explicit therapeutic plan, probably including initiation of somatic antidepressant treatment; in the majority of cases such treatment results in clinical improvement (Greenwald et al. 1989a; Nelson and Rosenberg 1991; Reifler et al. 1986). In contrast, it is unclear whether the fleeting affective symptoms to which Roth referred represent a true mood disorder and whether they either merit or respond to somatic antidepressant treatments.

Epidemiological Considerations

Depression in Dementia

A number of studies have addressed the prevalence of depression in dementia (Wragg and Jeste 1989). Unfortunately, there is tremendous inconsistency across studies, with prevalence rates ranging from 0% (Knesevich et al. 1983) to 86% (Merriam et al. 1988). Such a wide variation is at least in part ascribable to differences 1) across studies in differentiating depressive features, symptoms, and signs from a full-fledged major depressive episode or syndrome; 2) in patient samples (e.g., psychiatric versus nonpsychiatric dementia populations); and 3) in the application of specific diagnostic criteria (Burns 1990). The wide scatter also attests to the complexity and confusion encountered when considering a diagnosis of depression in a dementia patient. Nevertheless, an effort to distill the considerable prevalence literature reveals the following approximate breakdown:

- Major depression: 5%–15% of dementia patients (e.g., Greenwald et al. 1989a; Roth 1955; Rovner et al. 1989)
- Minor depression: 25% of dementia patients (e.g., Sultzer et al. 1992)
- Some depressive features: 50% of dementia patients (e.g., Cummings et al. 1987; Liston 1979; Sim and Sussman 1962)
- Family assessment of depression in their relative who has dementia: 50%–85% (e.g., MacKenzie et al. 1989; Merriam et al. 1988)

Depression in Alzheimer's Disease
Versus Multi-Infarct Dementia

The weight of studies that have examined the prevalence of depression in Alzheimer's dementia and multi-infarct dementia suggests a higher prevalence of major depression in multi-infarct dementia (20%–25%) (Cummings 1988; Cummings et al. 1987; Greenwald et al. 1989a) than in Alzheimer's disease (5%–15%) (Greenwald et al. 1989a; Roth 1955; Rovner et al. 1989). The increased prevalence in multi-infarct dementia is understandable in the context of an extensive literature linking ischemic cerebrovascular disease to affective illness (Parikh and Robinson 1987). For example, 30%–60% of stroke patients develop clinically significant depressions during the poststroke period (Lipsey et al. 1984), and more than 50% of stroke victims have been estimated to go on to develop multi-infarct dementia (Cummings 1987).

Depression in Mild, Moderate, and
Advanced Dementia

Although there is a widely held clinical view that depression more typically complicates early or mild dementia and is secondary to the experience and realization of cognitive loss, actual data supporting such a notion are less definitive. One study addressed the prevalence of a depressive syndrome among dementia patients with varying levels of cognitive deterioration; the authors reported that 33% of mildly impaired, 23% of moderately impaired, and 12% of severely impaired patients had depression (Reifler et al. 1982). In contrast, an examination of major depression in early Alzheimer's disease reported that 0% of 30 examinees were depressed (Knesevich et al. 1983). A study of patients with Alzheimer's disease and with multi-infarct dementia did report that in more severe Alzheimer's disease, depressed mood and scores on the Hamilton Rating Scale for Depression (HRSD) were lower, whereas in multi-infarct dementia such differences were negligible across the range of dementia severity (Fischer et al. 1990). The latter point is partially supported by findings of no significant relationship between dementia and depression severity (Cummings et al. 1987), with the caveat that no patient in this study who had obvious depression also had advanced dementia. On the other hand, an investigation of the prevalence of major depression in severe dementia patients living in special-care units for dementia in a nursing home reported a surprisingly high prevalence of depression (18% or 23%, depending on the criteria employed) (Greenwald and Kramer 1991). To some extent, these latter findings are buttressed by a recent report of an inverse correlation between scores on the HRSD and the Mini-Mental State Exam (MMSE) in patients with Alzheimer's dementia. That is, patients with more dementia (lower MMSE scores) had higher (worse) depression ratings (Sultzer et al. 1992). Taken together, these data suggest that clinicians should be sensitive to the fact that major depression can occur during all stages of dementia.

Depression in Nursing Home Residents With Dementia

Among nursing home residents, prevalence data indicate that approximately 40%–80% have dementia (Burns et al. 1988; Chandler and Chandler 1988; Rovner et al. 1986; Teeter et al. 1976) and 12% have major depression (Parmelee et al. 1989; Rovner et al. 1991). A significant proportion of nursing home residents have both dementia and depression (Parmelee et al. 1989; Rovner et al. 1986; Rovner et al. 1991). Major depression in this population is underdiagnosed and undertreated, associated with a higher mortality, and responsive to antidepressant therapy (Katz et al. 1990; Rovner et al. 1991).

Etiological Considerations

Depression complicating dementia has been described as typically occurring early in the course of intellectual deterioration, presumably secondary to the devastating psychological consequences of awareness of eroding cognitive capacities (Reifler et al. 1982). In fact, an extensive investigation and stimulating discussion about mood disturbance in "senile brain disease" (Miller 1980) noted that "a substantial number of case reports in the psychiatric literature" support the view that

> while depressive affect is either a common precursor of organic
> brain impairment or a concomitant of it at early subclinical
> stages, once the dementia has progressed to a diagnosable syn-
> drome, depressive behaviors tend to disappear and are replaced
> by blandness of affect and denial. (p. 106)

However, study data did not support this perspective: "the
clinical presence of dysphoric symptoms in even the most disoriented elderly subjects [i.e., those with the highest level of demen-
tia] in this study was striking." (p. 106)

Therefore, although it is clear that an early, reactive depression occurs in some individuals who are losing cognitive capacities, ample evidence exists that depression also occurs
throughout the course of dementia, in which case it seems less
plausible that the depression is a result simply of a psychological
adaptation to the awareness of cognitive and memory deterioration. In several case reports, individuals with moderate or even
severe dementia, whose condition had clearly progressed beyond the point of self-awareness, had a diagnosable major depression (DeMuth and Rand 1980; McAllister and Price 1982;
Shraberg 1978; Snow and Wells 1981). Hence, in contrast to psychological theories of Alzheimer's disease patients' depression,
there have emerged biological hypotheses about its etiopatho-
genesis, which are based on abnormalities in neuroanatomical
regions and neurotransmitters implicated in affective illness
(Whitehouse and Unnerstall 1988).

Coincident with early reports of locus coeruleus cell loss and
noradrenergic deficits in the brains of patients with Alzheimer's
disease (Bondareff et al. 1981; Mann et al. 1980; Perry et al. 1981;
Tomlinson et al. 1981; Yates et al. 1981), speculation arose that
such changes might underlie the existence of a depressive subgroup in those with Alzheimer's disease (K. L. Davis, personal
communication, 1981). The repeated demonstration of reductions in markers of neurotransmitters linked to the pathophysiology of depression stimulated additional conjecture on possible
noradrenergic and cholinergic etiologies of depression in Alzheimer's disease (Liston et al. 1987). The existence of serotonergic
deficiencies in Alzheimer's disease (e.g., Palmer et al. 1987; Procter et al. 1988; Yamamoto and Hirano 1985) further suggests that

abnormal serotonin neurotransmission may be important in the clinical expression of depression in this population (Lawlor 1990).

Several investigations lend data-based support to these ideas by comparing neurotransmitter-related brain markers in post-mortem studies of dementia patients with and without depression. Dementia patients with major depression had significantly more neurodegenerative findings in the noradrenergic locus coeruleus and dopaminergic substantia nigra than nondepressed counterparts with dementia (Zubenko and Moossy 1988). Similarly, Alzheimer's disease patients with depression had greater locus coeruleus neuronal loss than Alzheimer's disease patients without depression; a trend suggesting greater serotonergic dorsal raphe nucleus cell loss in depressed persons with dementia was also noted (Zweig et al. 1988).

Of related interest, in Parkinson's disease, cerebrospinal fluid levels of 5-hydroxyindoleacetic acid (5-HIAA), the major serotonin metabolite, were lower in depressed than in nondepressed patients (Mayeux et al. 1984) and lowest in patients with combined dementia and depression (Sano et al. 1989). A later study further corroborated the possible importance of the serotonin system in depression in Alzheimer's disease: it reported trend-level decrements in serotonin levels in the brains of depressed as compared with nondepressed Alzheimer's disease patients (Zubenko et al. 1990). However, in this study the major findings indicated a significant reduction in the level of norepinephrine in the cortex, with relative preservation of an acetylcholine marker, choline acetyltransferase (CAT) activity, in subcortical regions of the brains of depressed Alzheimer's disease patients. The investigators interpreted the CAT findings as suggesting that a threshold of remaining central cholinergic function was necessary for the expression of depression in individuals with dementia (Zubenko et al. 1990). This notion evokes the accumulated literature supporting cholinergic mediation of affective illness (summarized in Janowsky and Risch 1987). The concept of cholinergic mechanisms of affectivity in Alzheimer's disease is also indirectly supported by experiments demonstrating the provocation of overt depressive symptoms in Alzheimer's disease during cholinomimetic infusion trials (Davis et al. 1987; Molchan et al. 1991).

A possible unifying hypothesis to explain the diverse epidemiological reports on prevalence of depression in both mild and more severe Alzheimer's disease suggests that depression in Alzheimer's disease is expressed biphasically: there is an earlier, reactive component associated with awareness of cognitive decline; and there is a later, biologically determined depression, presumably based on decrements of neurotransmitters implicated in affective illness (Lawlor et al., unpublished data, cited in Sunderland et al. 1988a). Pathogenetic issues in depression complicating multi-infarct dementia have been less investigated than these issues in Alzheimer's disease. Neurochemical theories deriving largely from the poststroke depression literature suggest that depression in multi-infarct dementia is associated with left-sided, more frontal infarcts that interfere with ascending noradrenergic projections (Cummings 1988; Robinson and Starkstein 1990) and/or poststroke serotonergic dysregulation (Mayberg et al. 1988). There is also a growing database specifically implicating the basal ganglia in major depression (Baxter et al. 1985; Krishnan et al. 1992) and depression following stroke (Starkstein et al. 1988). Taken together, from a clinical standpoint the presence of lacunar infarcts of basal ganglia structures (particularly left-sided) on magnetic resonance imaging (MRI) or computed tomography (CT) scans of multi-infarct dementia patients could suggest a greater susceptibility to developing depression, help validate a clinical diagnosis of depression, and contribute to the clinician's decision to initiate antidepressant treatment.

Other relevant issues in considering causes of depression in multi-infarct dementia include the degree of morbidity/disability associated with both cerebrovascular insults and related arteriosclerotic cardiovascular disease (e.g., myocardial infarction, angina, claudication), the possible contributions to depression of centrally active cardiovascular medications, a personal history of depression, and a family history of depression (Cummings 1988). Regarding this last point, depression in Alzheimer's disease dementia has been associated with a greater frequency of depression in first-degree family members (Pearlson et al. 1990). This association suggests that depression in Alzheimer's disease may be determined in part by genetic predisposition. Hence a family history of depression may be an important clinical clue in supporting a diagnosis of major depression in a patient with

Alzheimer's disease in whom depression is suspected but not certain.

Clinical Diagnosis

Over the past decade there have appeared an impressive array of experimental and clinical reports about depression complicating dementia, from which an aggregate clinical wisdom about diagnosis and phenomenology can be derived. In this section, key clinically useful observations are discussed, followed by illustrative case vignettes.

Overlap of Symptoms of Dementia and Depression

The diagnosis of depression in an individual who already has dementia can be especially vexing, because several symptoms of dementia and depression overlap. Appetite disturbance, weight loss, sleep disturbance, psychomotor changes, diminished interest, social withdrawal, increased emotionality, and cognitive changes all occur in each of the dementia and depression syndromes. In one study, in fact, symptoms of major depression significantly correlated with an increasing severity of dementia in Alzheimer's disease patients in whom experienced clinicians had excluded a major depression (Greenwald et al. 1986a). The authors concluded that major depressive symptoms (but not necessarily a major depressive *syndrome*) are part and parcel of the Alzheimer's disease syndrome. This perspective is supported by recent data reporting that scores on the HRSD—possibly weighted by neurovegetative overlap items—are higher in patients with advanced Alzheimer's disease, but that these symptoms may actually be unrelated to a mood disorder; rather, they may reflect advancing dementia-related disability (Sultzer et al. 1992). Another study (Rubin and Kinscherf 1989), dealing with patients with very mild Alzheimer's disease without major depression, found the presence of compromised interest, concentration, and energy and psychomotor changes. The presence of these symptoms similarly suggested that they were a result of the process of Alzheimer's disease, not representative of a concurrent depression. With this in mind, how can the clinician interpret overlapping symptoms and signs like appetite and sleep disturbance, psychomotor changes, and aspontaneity in considering the diagnosis of major depression in a dementia patient?

To discern major depression in dementia, the nature and quality of depressive features have to be carefully considered. Rather than evaluate the mere presence of depressive symptoms, clinicians must determine whether there has been a *change* in these symptoms. For example, a patient with moderate dementia who consistently eats less than during the predementia period now practically stops eating and loses 10 pounds over a 6-week period. Or a dementia patient who wandered aimlessly but could be redirected to activities now paces unrelentingly and cannot be refocused. These examples illustrate a clear-cut acute or subacute *change* in previously present depressionlike symptoms (appetite disturbance and psychomotor agitation, respectively) and suggest that some degree of investigative interviewing—often of multiple informants (family members/caregivers at home; nurses and aides in nursing homes)—may be necessary for clarifying the presence of depressive symptoms. These kinds of changes should increase the clinician's suspicion that a major depression has developed. The relatively new depression scales designed specifically for use in dementia patients (Alexopoulos et al. 1988; Sunderland et al. 1988b) incorporate the concept of change in (rather than just the presence of) vegetative symptoms into the rating of depression in dementia patients. Conventional geriatric depression scales may have limited applicability in dementia patients (Burke et al. 1989).

Because neurovegetative symptoms are common in nondepressed dementia patients, an additional suggestion is that the clinician focus on intrapsychic features of depression (Lazarus et al. 1987)—like hopelessness, helplessness, worthlessness, worry, and despair—during the diagnostic assessment for depression. According to this view, the presence of such intrapsychic depressive phenomena carries more weight in diagnosing depression in dementia than the presence of overlapping vegetative symptoms.

Focus on Signs Rather Than Symptoms

Because of often-impaired comprehension and communicative capacity in dementia, it may be necessary to concentrate on signs rather than symptoms when diagnosing depression in a dementia patient. This was recognized in one of the earlier attempts to develop a rating scale for depression in dementia patients—the Depressive Signs Scale, which identifies and rates observable rather than elicitable features of depression (Katona and Aldridge 1985). Features of this scale include sad appearance, reactivity of sad appearance, agitation in the daytime, slowness of movement, slowness of speech, early waking, loss of appetite, diurnal variation in mood (mornings worst), and interest in surroundings.

The concept of relying on signs rather than symptoms has a particular application in identifying depression in advanced dementia patients, who are often unreliable informants, hardly communicative, or even mute and nonresponsive. To enhance assessment in such patients, a gestalt rating of depression for advanced dementia was developed and evaluated on a special-care unit for residents with severe dementia in a nursing home (Greenwald and Kramer 1991). Operationalized criteria for depression in advanced dementia include the following:

1. The prominent presence of one or more of the following features in a nondelirious patient:
   a) Lack of environmental reactivity in an otherwise interactive person
   b) Affective anxiety (anxiety in the context of tearfulness, worry, frantic but incomprehensible efforts at communication)
   c) Beseeching quality (importuning for help, clutching at interviewer in a help-seeking manner)
   d) Depressed appearance (e.g., weepiness)
   e) Affect-laden psychomotor agitation; for example, hand-wringing, pacing with a worried expression, angst-ridden self-abusive behaviors such as
      • Hair pulling
      • Picking at self
      • Banging
      • Screaming either with a depressive content (e.g., "Help me, help me, help me" or "I'm no good, I'm no good, I'm no good") or with an anxious, worried, or suffering tone (e.g., "Aaahhhhhh!!!!" or "Noooooooooo!!!")

2. Depressive feature(s) prominent enough to warrant a somatic antidepressant treatment trial, in the opinion of an experienced geriatric psychiatrist or psychologist.

The gestalt rating identified 23% of 74 patients with severe dementia as depressed; the rating had a high interrater reliability (kappa coefficient = .88) among experienced geropsychiatric clinicians. Furthermore, in patients ratable by more conventional assessments (only half of the sample), gestalt ratings had a concordance of more than 90% with major depression as described in DSM-III-R (American Psychiatric Association 1987). Of additional interest was the finding that among an array of standardized ratings by nurses, only the nurse rating of depressed appearance correlated with the experienced-clinician rating of major depression. This suggests that the simple assessment by nursing home nurses of whether a familiar resident with advanced dementia looks depressed may have some validity in identifying heretofore underrecognized concomitant major depression.

Does a Depressive Syndrome in Dementia Have Unique Features?

The identification of depression in a dementia patient would be aided by the presence of a unique or characteristic clinical profile. For example, some evidence exists suggesting that, when compared with younger depressed individuals, depression in elderly people without dementia is characterized by more somatic and hypochondriacal complaints, greater delusionality, and more frequent depression-dependent cognitive impairment (Folstein and McHugh 1978; Meyers and Greenberg 1986; Sunderland et al. 1988a). However, systematic efforts to identify a unique symptom complex in depression complicating dementia have not been fruitful.

One study (Greenwald et al. 1989a) employed more than 50 items reflecting depressive symptomatology from the Schedule for Affective Disorders and Schizophrenia (SADS) and the Present State Examination (PSE). The study compared clinical phenomenology in patients with mostly mild to moderate depression, elderly depressed patients without dementia, and non-depressed control subjects with dementia. For the most part, symptom profiles were similar between the age-matched group with dementia and depression and the group with depression only. Only the items "rejection sensitivity" and "self-pity" differentiated the group with dementia and depression from the group with depression only. The authors concluded that the symptom profile of depression complicating dementia is largely similar to depression in elderly people without dementia. These findings are similar to results from descriptive studies of poststroke depression (Lipsey et al. 1986), depression associated with Parkinson's disease (Mayeux et al. 1986), and depression in brain injury (McAllister et al. 1988).

Taken together, these studies suggest that despite underlying brain disease, the phenomenological expression of depression is usually predictable. However, clinicians must bear in mind that several uncontrolled clinical and case reports call attention to unusual or atypical presentations of depression in dementia (DeMuth and Rand 1980; McAllister and Price 1982; Shraberg 1978; Snow and Wells 1981), wherein somatic antidepressant treatment was associated with obvious improvement. This is especially true in patients with advanced dementia, in whom severely agitated behaviors like screaming, banging, or self-abusive actions have been interpreted as a possible forme fruste of major depression (Greenwald et al. 1986b). A relationship between verbal agitation in dementia and depressed affect has been identified in nursing home residents with dementia (Cohen-Mansfield and Marx 1988).

One additional note: in the above-described study comparing patients who had dementia and depression, depression only, and dementia only (Greenwald et al. 1989a), only the patients with dementia and depression or with depression only manifested mood-congruent depressive delusions (that is, delusions consistent with a depressive theme—e.g., delusions of impoverishment, guilt or sin, disease, nihilism). No dementia-only patient had mood-congruent delusions. Although sample sizes were small, and differences did not reach statistical significance, these data imply that the presence of mood-congruent affective delusions in dementia suggests major depression.

Cognitive Changes Secondary to Depression

Major depression, especially in elderly people, may be accompanied by reversible cognitive changes (Cohen et al. 1982; Sternberg and Jarvik 1976). This phenomenon has variably been called dementia syndrome of depression (Folstein and McHugh 1978), cognitive impairment of depression (Reifler 1982), and depressive pseudodementia (McAllister 1983). Approximately 20%–30% of elderly patients with major depression manifest cognitive changes that improve coincident with improvement in the underlying depression (Greenwald et al. 1989b; LaRue et al. 1986; Post 1966). There is no reason to assume that elderly dementia patients with major depression are not susceptible to the development of a depressive, state-dependent cognitive worsening. In fact, data exist documenting that cognitive impairment (including functional abilities) in depressed patients with dementia, as measured by structured brief cognitive rating scales, improves after successful antidepressant treatment, even though overall cognitive function remains in the range of marked dementia (Greenwald et al. 1989a). Furthermore, a study of instrumental activities of daily living and depression in Alzheimer's disease suggested that depression exerts a suppressive effect on functional status (Pearson et al. 1989). In contrast, a neuropsychological nontreatment study of Alzheimer's disease patients with and without depression reported no difference in neuropsychological deficits between groups at baseline and at 1-year follow-up; the authors concluded that depression does not appear to modify the neuropsychological features or the rate of progression of Alzheimer's disease (Lopez et al. 1990). One of the only controlled treatment studies of depression in Alzheimer's disease (Reifler et al. 1989) reported controversial findings in terms of antidepressant benefit to cognitive functioning.

Subcortical dementia is a term used to describe neurological and behavioral phenomena associated with neurodegenerative disorders affecting subcortical brain structures. Examples of conditions (and the underlying area of brain pathology) associated with subcortical dementia include Parkinson's disease (substantia nigra), Huntington's disease (caudate), progressive supranuclear palsy (midbrain), and lacunar state (basal ganglia).

Neurological features of subcortical dementia include unsteady, ataxic gait; tremor; dyskinesia; hypophonia; mutism; and stooped posture. Behavioral phenomena include psychomotor retardation; slowing of thought, comprehension, and verbalization; forgetfulness; apathy; and decreased drive (Benson 1983). The neuropsychological profile of "depressive pseudodementia" has been described as subcortical, characterized by aspontaneity and diminished effort and initiative (Caine 1981). Hence, the development of obvious subcortical-like phenomena—apathy, aspontaneity, bradyphrenia, and diminished initiative and effort—in a previously energetic and motivated Alzheimer's disease patient might be a clinical clue that depression has developed.

Admittedly, the identification of worsened cognitive performance secondary to depression in an individual with dementia at best is challenging and at worst requires extraordinary clinical acumen, because such changes may become embedded in an impression of global cognitive deterioration and may hardly be evident. However, in some patients, especially those with early Alzheimer's disease, even subtle cognitive changes may be readily recognizable. Recently developed cognitive worsening in dementia patients, therefore—especially subcortical-like changes—should cause the clinician to consider the possibility of major depression.

Medical History

The presence of dementia does not confer immunity against having, or having had, other medical and/or psychiatric illnesses. Hence, as is true for all patients—especially the elderly—a comprehensive medical assessment and current medication review is required when evaluating a dementia patient for the possibility of depression (Cummings 1988). Depression-related conditions like cancer, hypothyroidism, hypercalcemia, and vitamin deficiencies must be ruled out. Medications linked to depression—including antihypertensives, sedative-hypnotics, and cardiac and pulmonary medications—may have to be changed, discontinued, or dose-adjusted.

Personal and Family History of Depression

Not to be overlooked in assessing depression in dementia patients is a personal history of depression in the patient or a family history of affective illness in a relative. The study cited above (Pearlson et al. 1990) found that depressed Alzheimer's disease patients had a significantly greater frequency of first-degree relatives with depression than did nondepressed Alzheimer's disease patients. A comparison of psychiatric history between Alzheimer's disease patients and age-matched control subjects without dementia found that Alzheimer's disease patients had a significantly greater likelihood of psychiatric morbidity earlier in life; unipolar depression and paranoid disorder were the most common diagnoses (Agbayewa 1986).

Laboratory Diagnosis of Depression in Dementia

There is currently no consistent laboratory tool to diagnose either depression or depression in dementia. During the heyday of interest in the dexamethasone suppression test (DST) as a biological probe to detect depression, several studies employed the DST in Alzheimer's disease. Significant proportions (at times more than 50%) of nondepressed Alzheimer's disease patients had abnormal DST results, suggesting that the utility of this procedure in diagnosing depression in Alzheimer's disease was limited (Greenwald et al. 1986a; Raskind et al. 1982; Spar and Gerner 1982). However, one investigation did demonstrate a relationship between 8:00 A.M. postdexamethasone cortisol levels and endogenous depressive symptoms (Greenwald et al. 1986a), although the sample of Alzheimer's disease patients studied excluded patients with a syndrome of major depression. An investigation of the DST in depressed and nondepressed dementia patients found abnormal DSTs only in dementia patients who also met criteria for depression (Carnes et al. 1983). Another report suggested that the DST was probably of little use in identifying depression in patients with moderate or severe dementia but that it might be useful for recognizing depression in patients with mild impairment (Jenike and Albert 1984).

Interestingly, a clinical report presenting a longitudinal case study of a patient with dementia and depression demonstrated continued reversal of an abnormal DST following antidepressant therapy (Wamboldt et al. 1985). Another brief report also documented normalizing of the DST in several dementia patients while they were taking antidepressants (Moffatt 1984). However, caution was subsequently urged in assuming that the antidepressant action of the drugs was responsible for reversion of the DST to normal (Mahendra 1985). Taken together, these data suggest that the DST probably has limited application in the discrimination of depression in Alzheimer's disease, but that in some patients it could have a role as a biological validator of antidepressant response.

Discriminant function analyses of electroencephalographic (EEG) sleep data in elderly persons with dementia and depression reliably distinguish depressed patients without dementia from dementia patients with depressive features (Reynolds et al. 1988). Furthermore, mixed-symptom patients in this study (either "dementia syndrome of depression" or "primary degenerative dementia with depressive features") were correctly classified 64% of the time. However, the investigation did not explicitly address sleep laboratory differentiation of dementia patients with and without depression.

DSM Nomenclature

As has been aptly noted (Burns 1989), the DSM-III-R criteria do not allow the dual diagnosis of dementia and major depressive episode. Therefore, by current DSM-III-R criteria, an elderly patient presenting with an unequivocal preexisting dementia of the Alzheimer type of a few years' duration, who has subsequently developed a superimposed major depression, should be categorized as 290.21: primary degenerative dementia of the Alzheimer type, senile onset, *with depression* (italics added). However, explicit criteria for the modifier *with depression* are not identified in DSM-III-R.

DSM-IV (American Psychiatric Association 1994) modified the dementia nomenclature; therefore, the patient described above would now be categorized as 290.21: dementia of the Alzheimer's type, late onset, with depressed mood. In DSM-IV the modifier *depressed mood* is explained as follows: "if depressed mood (including presentations that meet full symptom criteria for a Major Depressive Episode) is the predominant feature." (p. 143) Both DSM-III-R and DSM-IV categorizations could apply to dementia patients with either subsyndromal depressive features or a major depressive episode. DSM-IV advances the distinction somewhat by necessitating that "depressed mood" be "the predominant feature." However, to encourage greater diagnostic consistency across centers and published reports and in treatment trials, a useful classification might be that the modifier *with depressed mood* be further modified to either "with major depressive episode or *with minor or transient depressive features.*

Case 1

Mr. A, an 88-year-old widower, experienced progressive forgetfulness over a period of approximately 2 years. He complained bitterly that he was "not right"; according to family and friends, over the past 4–6 months he had been despondent and irritable over his diminishing independence and competence. Intermittent tearfulness, reduced appetite, and bowel preoccupation were noted. Mr. A's internist had treated him for depression with several antidepressants, some in combination with a neuroleptic, without significant improvement. A mental status examination revealed a constricted affect and sad mood, a statement about welcoming death but no suicidal ideation, guilt feelings about past mistakes, self-deprecation and decreased self-esteem ("I have little to offer others"), diminished interest in the news and in social gatherings, anergia and anhedonia, severe constipation, indecision, rumination, worry, suspiciousness, and sleep disturbance. A cognitive examination revealed deficits in orientation, attention, calculation, recall, and topographical orientation, as well as impoverishment of vocabulary, naming and word-finding problems, paraphasic errors, occasional accidents in the bathroom, sloppy eating, and difficulty in dressing.

Mr. A was painfully aware of his cognitive deficits and his mood state ("I feel morbid"). The Mini-Mental State Exam (MMSE) score was 20/30. Family history was noteworthy for probable depression in the patient's mother and brother. Mr. A was hospitalized. A complete dementia workup did not reveal any reversible etiology. A diagnosis of primary degenerative dementia of the Alzheimer's type, senile onset, with concomitant major depression, was made. Two additional antidepressant treatment trials failed, and ECT was broached; however, the patient and family were adamant in their refusal to consider ECT.

Over the next 2 weeks the patient developed increased irritability, suspiciousness, restlessness, and psychomotor agitation (pacing incessantly). He became delusional about bowel disease, felt hopeless, and repeatedly stated "I'm in trouble." On reexamination his MMSE decreased to 16/30, and he had lost 4 pounds. Following the family's reluctant acquiescence, Mr. A began treatment with ECT for suspected delusional depression superimposed on a preexisting Alzheimer's dementia. He received five nondominant, unilateral, pulse-wave ECT treatments without any benefit. He was switched to bilateral ECT and after the second treatment manifested obvious improvement. Mr. A received a total of six bilateral ECT treatments and showed dramatic improvement in his depressive symptoms. Following completion of his ECT, a repeat MMSE score was 24/30. Lithium was titrated up to 450 mg, with a blood level of 0.6 mEq/L, for prophylaxis of depression. He was discharged at his request to a health-related facility, and he has remained on lithium without recurrence of major depression.

Points of Relevance in Case 1

1. *Typical depressive symptoms.*   In this patient with dementia, the depressive syndrome presented with classic depressive symptoms and mood-congruent ideas that evolved to delusions.

2. *Improvement in cognitive function with successful somatic treatment of depression.*   The MMSE score was 20/30 on admission; as depression worsened, the MMSE score decreased to 16/30. Following ECT, the MMSE score improved to 24/30. This score—and Mr. A's overall posttreatment behavior and functioning—remained consistent with a diagnosis of underlying dementia; however, it represented a 50% improvement over his lowest MMSE score.

3. *Family history of depression.*   The patient's mother and brother had a history of apparent major depression.

Case 2

Mr. B, a successful 66-year-old active architect, presented with complaints of 1–2 years of slight forgetfulness and mistakes in business that befuddled him. A complete organic workup was negative in terms of medical or neurological etiology of cognitive changes. However, a neuropsychological battery revealed delayed verbal and visual recall deficits, mild naming problems, decreased verbal fluency, and significant word-finding difficulty in spontaneous speech consistent with early-stage Alzheimer's disease. Mr. B and his wife requested a frank discussion of the findings. The possibility of Alzheimer's disease was raised and obviously unsettled Mr. B. He quickly volunteered that, ethically, he should immediately phase himself out of active architectural work and hasten his upcoming planned retirement. Although the weight of that decision was apparent, Mr. B joked that he could devote himself increasingly to golf.

Over the next several months, Mr. and Mrs. B reported subtle diminution in Mr. B's animation. Despite Mr. B's continuing consultatory relationship to his firm, Mrs. B expressed concern that since his diagnosis, Mr. B was becoming increasingly socially isolated and had lost all interest in sex. He said that he was becoming a burden to his wife. She noted that he also had a lowered threshold for emotionality. For example, at the funeral of an acquaintance, he sobbed out of proportion to the personal loss that the death represented. On the other hand, he continued to enjoy golf, ate heartily, slept as before, and expressed interest and excitement in a long-planned trip to France.

A diagnosis of possible concomitant major depression was made. Initial antidepressant therapy with nortriptyline was discontinued secondary to hypotension, and fluoxetine was begun. After approximately 3.5 weeks of treatment with 20 mg of fluoxetine daily, Mr. B demonstrated reduced emotional lability and an improved mood and outlook. Mr. B then requested some form of "talking therapy." Adjunctive supportive-educational psychotherapy was initiated, and the patient was able to articulate his future fears and his at times unrealistic expectations about Alzheimer's disease. Combined pharmacotherapy and psychotherapy resulted in improved mood, socialization, interests, enjoyment, and libido (with a return of intimate involvement with his wife) and a greater understanding of what to anticipate in terms of Alzheimer's disease progression.

Points of Relevance in Case 2

1. *Reactive depression.* Dysphoric symptomatology clearly developed as a reaction to the patient's realization that his symptoms probably represented Alzheimer's disease.
2. *Equivocal nature of syndromal diagnosis of depression.* Although several features of depression were present, Mr. B also maintained his appetite, had no sleep disturbance, and continued to enjoy his work and avocations. Nevertheless, a constellation of signs and symptoms—including hyperemotionality, loss of libido, decreased self-esteem, and diminished vivacity—suggested a diagnosis of depression.

Case 3

Mr. C, an 83-year-old retired musician, was referred for evaluation of abnormal behaviors. His medical history included poorly defined neuroretinitis, which had forced a premature retirement secondary to near blindness; hypertension; and mild renal insufficiency. He had been diagnosed approximately 1–2 years earlier with a mild to moderate degree of "senility" by his long-time internist—without a comprehensive workup, however. Mr. C had a questionable history of depression, secondary to treatment of hypertension with reserpine many years earlier; he had been ultimately treated with ECT, with limited success. Over the past 6–8 weeks, Mr. C had developed a worsening behavioral picture characterized by intermittent agitation (e.g., fidgeting, constantly calling his wife), noticeable apathy about issues he had previously been more interested in, and reduction in his usual sense of humor.

On examination, a brief cognitive screen revealed marked deficits in orientation, attention, and recent and remote memory. On an MMSE (modified because of his visual impairment), Mr. C scored 11 out of a possible 27 points. He was hospitalized for further workup and treatment. A comprehensive dementia assessment revealed multiple small infarcts involving the lateral portion of the basal ganglia bilaterally on computed tomography (CT) scan. The mental status examination was significant for occasional weepiness, decreased appetite, unfounded concerns about his wife's infidelity and about the likelihood of impending impoverishment, moaning as if in physical discomfort yet without somatic localization, and exaggerated feelings of helplessness.

A diagnosis of multi-infarct dementia with likely superimposed major depression was made. A tricyclic trial was interrupted by the development of urinary retention, and tranylcypromine provoked a rash. Phenelzine was initiated and titrated successfully to 45 mg/day. Mr. C's affective symptomatology gradually improved, then abated. He continued to display obvious dementia but was discharged in a behaviorally stable condition to home.

Points of Relevance in Case 3

1. *Basal ganglia lesions on CT scan.* Neuroimaging identification of basal ganglia infarcts, especially left-sided lesions, during workup should suggest to the clinician a possible predisposition to depression. In a study of single basal ganglia infarcts and poststroke depression, 88% of patients with left basal ganglia lesions were depressed (Starkstein et al. 1988). Furthermore, preexisting subcortical disease may be associated with geriatric depression (Coffey et al. 1990) and may increase the risk of developing major depression following stroke (Robinson and Starkstein 1990).
2. *Personal history of depression.* Mr. C had once experienced a major depression severe enough to warrant a trial of ECT.
3. *Moaning as an atypical depressive symptom.* Reports of depression complicating moderate to severe dementia describe unusual, often verbally agitated behaviors as possibly representing an idiosyncratic expression of depression (Cohen-Mansfield and Marx 1988; DeMuth and Rand 1980; Greenwald and Kramer 1991; Greenwald et al. 1986b).
4. *Mood-congruent symptomatology in suggesting major depression.* In this case, the presence of mood-congruent ideation and delusionality regarding infidelity and impoverishment support a diagnosis of major depression.

Case 4

Mrs. D, a 78-year-old widow, was institutionalized in a nursing home following her second stroke, which left her both physically and cognitively compromised. Over a 3-year period, Mrs. D developed advanced dementia, was chairbound, and was doubly incontinent. She had periods of near mutism alternating with periods of loquaciousness of a practically unintelligible nature that often evolved into utterance of profanities at passersby. During the past several months, she had been observed to laugh and cry uncontrollably and almost grotesquely and had been noted to be increasingly irritable. When approached, Mrs. D grabbed staff in a beseeching manner and cried "help, help, help, help, help" with increasing loudness, culminating in a shriek that was described by the ward charge nurse as sounding "as if she was being tortured." According to night shift nursing notes, her sleep, which had typically been disrupted during the night, was now also characterized by difficulty in falling asleep, which had heretofore not been an obvious problem. A complete medical workup revealed a questionable urinary tract infection, which quickly resolved with antibiotic treatment; the behaviors, however, persisted.

The patient, who had previously allowed herself to be made up by the staff and visit the facility hairdresser, now was resistant and looked disheveled, unkempt, and worried. A nurse's aide commented, "She's got a filthy mouth, but now she seems so sad." Her family, alarmed by the change in her behavior, requested a geropsychiatric consultation after her regular house doctor had attempted to prescribe an antipsychotic.

A provisional diagnosis of major depression and intermittent pathological hyperemotionality complicating advanced multi-infarct dementia was made. Reluctance to give a drug with any appreciable anticholinergic properties precluded prescribing a tricyclic antidepressant, and the family refused a monoamine oxidase inhibitor upon hearing about the possibility of a hypertensive crisis. A trial of trazodone was initiated. The dose was gradually titrated up to 350 mg/day; the only significant side effect was peripheral leg edema. Profane outbursts, irritability, pathological emotionality, and related verbal-vocal agitation gradually subsided; cooperativeness increased.

Points of Relevance in Case 4

1. *Interpretation of agitated behaviors.* Many of this patient's agitated features could be interpreted as "depressive equiva-

lents": profane outbursts as a form of irritability/hostility,
screaming for help as a form of helplessness, and shrieking as
a form of psychic anguish.

2. *Pathological emotionality.* Pathological weepiness and laugh-
ter can be associated with poststroke syndromes and cortical
dementias (Kaufman 1981). The demonstrated responsive-
ness of hyperemotionality to antidepressants suggests a possible relationship with depression (Schiffer et al. 1985).

3. *Depression in advanced dementia.* Major depression can occur
in patients with advanced dementia, however obscured by
late-stage cognitive incapacity and marked behavioral disturbances. Although Mrs. D was incapable of responding to
questions about depression or of articulating depressive
complaints, observable signs (irritability, angst-laden verbal
outbursts, weepiness, depressed appearance, lack of reaction
to presumed formerly pleasurable activities, change in sleep
patterns) suggested affective disorder.

Case 5

Mrs. E, an 86-year-old widow, was referred for "depression"
characterized by apathy, diminished alertness and attention,
crying periods, loss of appetite, sleep disturbance, and lightheadedness. Her medical history was significant for hypertension, angina, congestive heart failure, vertigo, degenerative joint
disease, cataracts, and questionable "seizures" characterized by
"blankness and mumbling." Careful history taking from family
members revealed a likely several-year diagnosis of dementia,
which had been worked up by a local neurologist and included
relevant blood tests, a CT scan of the head, and an EEG. The EEG
revealed right frontotemporal slowing. Although the CT scan
did not reveal any infarcts, Mrs. E's history suggested the presence of risk factors for multi-infarct dementia, and she was given
a provisional diagnosis of a mixed Alzheimer's disease–multi-
infarct dementia. The family minimized the importance of this
diagnosis, stating that Mrs. E was old and emphasizing that the
key issue was her depression.

On examination, Mrs. E was a pleasant and cooperative
woman who smiled graciously and attempted to be accommo-
dating during cognitive testing. Her MMSE score was 18/30.

During the interview Mrs. E sporadically cried on occasions seemingly unrelated to content, and there were periods when she was aspontaneous, with a long latency in responding to questions. She had lost weight and indicated that food "does not taste the same to me." Mrs. E also dozed off repeatedly during the interview, then apologized. On occasion, her voice trailed off and became almost inaudible, with jumbled words. Medications included propranolol, isosorbide dinitrate, dipyridamole, sulindac, aspirin, alprazolam, transdermal nitroglycerine, and phenobarbital. The patient was hospitalized on a geriatric psychiatry unit for observation and further workup. Despite the family's protestations that Mrs. E was obviously depressed, the mental health staff did not have the impression of pervasive depression. During the day, especially during activities, the patient was usually pleasant, cooperative, and friendly, albeit confused.

The staff reported that during the night Mrs. E's confusion worsened and she was often observed to be talking to herself in her room. Review of the original indications and reasons for continuing the use of propranolol, dipyridamole, sulindac, alprazolam, transdermal nitroglycerine, and phenobarbital suggested that all these medications could be discontinued. A provisional diagnosis of cumulative medication-induced delirium was made, with fluctuating associated affectivity. Over a 2-month period all medications except isosorbide dinitrate and aspirin were gradually decreased and discontinued. During this time, behavioral symptoms slowly yet obviously subsided. Cognitive ratings also improved, although evidence of significant underlying impairment remained.

Points of Relevance in Case 5

1. *Considering delirium or medication effects in behaviorally disturbed dementia patients.* In elderly patients, delirium can commonly masquerade as depression (Lipowski 1989). Furthermore, brain disease is a risk factor for delirium (Berezin 1985); hence elderly dementia patients are especially vulnerable. Polypharmacy is also common in elderly patients. Therefore, before an antidepressant (or any psychotropic) drug is begun with a geriatric patient who has dementia, all medications should be reviewed. When possible, unneces-

sary drugs should be discontinued, regimens simplified, and dosages reduced. In Mrs. E's case, several of the medication classes she was taking have depressogenic potential. These include beta-blockers, barbiturates, and benzodiazepines. On geriatric psychiatry inpatient units, one of the most successful "treatments" for behavioral disturbance in dementia is discontinuation of unnecessary centrally active medications.

2. *Overdiagnosis of depression by family members in their relatives who have dementia.* At least two studies provide data that depression in dementia is probably overdiagnosed by family members. One survey reported an unrealistically high 86% prevalence of depression according to family members' assessment (Merriam et al. 1988); another investigation found that family members diagnosed depression in 50% of their relatives who had dementia, whereas a mental health professional found a prevalence of only 14% in the same population (MacKenzie et al. 1989). Because of the significant incidence of depression among caregivers of dementia patients, a contagion effect has been suggested, wherein depression in one person may be associated with depression in the other (Truax and Teri 1990). Therefore, although family input is essential in obtaining a comprehensive geropsychiatric assessment, clinicians should not rely solely on family/caregiver evaluations of depression. In the case of Mrs. E, it appeared that depression was a more acceptable diagnosis for her family than confusion or intellectual impairment.

3. *Depressive symptoms that are transient and not sustained.* Affective symptoms in Mrs. E were not pervasive. Most of the time, Mrs. E was pleasant and cooperative. Such fleeting affectivity suggests that a major depressive *syndrome* may *not* be present.

Summary and Conclusions

The recognition of a major depressive syndrome in a dementia patient is at times obvious: most dementia patients when depressed manifest a characteristic depressive syndrome. However, the presentation of depression in dementia (particularly in more advanced illness) can also be atypical. In such cases, identification of depression requires both diagnostic foresight (i.e., anticipating that a treatable major depression may be present) and phenomenological perspicacity (discerning the trees of likely depressive features from the blurry forest of cognitive-behavioral aberrancy). With this in mind, clinical indicators that may help identify depression in dementia include the following:

- Acute or subacute worsening of cognitive and instrumental impairment, especially if characterized by diminished initiative, spontaneity, and motivation (so-called subcortical behavioral features)
- Change in, rather than the mere presence of, neurovegetative symptoms like sleep and appetite disturbance
- Prominent intrapsychic symptoms of depression, including hopelessness, helplessness, and worthlessness
- The presence of mood-congruent depressive ideation, delusions, or hallucinations
- Affective coloring of severe agitated behaviors, like incessant screaming and pacing or self-abusive actions
- Personal history of depression
- Family history of depression

Neuroimaging findings of basal ganglia infarction, especially left-sided, suggest that a brain substrate possibly predisposing to depression may be present (Robinson and Starkstein 1990; Starkstein et al. 1988).

Finally, it is important to remember that patients with dementia still confront the same emotion-filled trials that challenge healthy elderly people: too frequent illnesses and deaths of beloved contemporaries, societal ostracism, neglectful children, physical frailties, financial instability, and reluctant and bewildering relocations. In evaluating and treating depression in dementia patients, this context should not be overlooked.

References

Agbayewa MO: Earlier psychiatric morbidity in patients with Alzheimer's disease. J Am Geriatr Soc 34:561–564, 1986

Alexopoulos GS, Abrams RC, Young RC, et al: Cornell Scale for depression in dementia. Biol Psychiatry 23:271–284, 1988

American Psychiatric Association: Diagnostic and Statistical Manual of Mental Disorders, 3rd Edition, Revised. Washington, DC, American Psychiatric Association, 1987

American Psychiatric Association: Diagnostic and Statistical Manual of Mental Disorders, 4th Edition. Washington, DC, American Psychiatric Association, 1994

Baxter LR, Phelps ME, Mazziotta JC, et al: Cerebral metabolic rates for glucose in mood disorders studied with positron emission tomography (PET) and (F-18)-fluoro-2-deoxyglucose (FDG). Arch Gen Psychiatry 42:441–447, 1985

Benson DF: Subcortical dementia: a clinical approach, in The Dementias. Edited by Mayeux R, Rosen WG. New York, Raven, 1983, pp 185–194

Berezin EV: Delirium in the elderly: assessment and management (Clinical Perspectives on Aging series, Monograph No. 3). Philadelphia, PA, Wyeth Laboratories, 1985

Bleuler EP: Lehrbuch der Psychiatrie. Berlin, 1923. Translated as Textbook of Psychiatry by Brill AA. New York, Macmillan, 1924

Bondareff W, Mountjoy CQ, Roth M: Selective loss of neurones of origin of adrenergic projection to cerebral cortex (nucleus locus coeruleus) in senile dementia. Lancet 1:783–784, 1981

Burke WJ, Houston MJ, Boust SJ, et al: Use of the Geriatric Depression Scale in dementia of the Alzheimer type. J Am Geriatr Soc 37:856–860, 1989

Burns A: Disorders of affect in Alzheimer's disease. International Journal of Geriatric Psychiatry 5:63–66, 1990

Burns BJ, Larson DB, Goldstrom ID, et al: Mental disorder among nursing home patients: preliminary findings from the national nursing home survey pretest. International Journal of Geriatric Psychiatry 3:27–35, 1988

Caine ED: Pseudodementia: current concepts and future directions. Arch Gen Psychiatry 38:1359–1364, 1981

Carnes M, Smith JC, Kalin NH, et al: The dexamethasone suppression test in demented outpatients with and without depression. Psychiatry Res 9:337–344, 1983

Chandler JD, Chandler JE: The prevalence of neuropsychiatric disorders in a nursing home population. J Geriatr Psychiatry Neurol 1:71–76, 1988

Coffey CE, Figiel GS, Djang WT, et al: Subcortical hyperintensity on magnetic resonance imaging: a comparison of normal and depressed elderly subjects. Am J Psychiatry 147:187–189, 1990

Cohen RM, Weingartner HW, Smallberg SA, et al: Effort and cognition in depression. Arch Gen Psychiatry 39:593–597, 1982

Cohen-Mansfield J, Marx MS: Relationship between depression and agitation in nursing home residents. Comprehensive Gerontology B2:141–146, 1988

Cole JO, Branconnier R, Salomon M, et al: Tricyclic use in the cognitively impaired elderly. J Clin Psychiatry 44:14–19, 1983

Cummings JL: Multi-infarct dementia: diagnosis and management. Psychosomatics 28:117–126, 1987

Cummings JL: Depression in vascular dementia. Hillside Journal of Clinical Psychiatry 10:209–231, 1988

Cummings JL, Miller B, Hill MA, et al: Neuropsychiatric aspects of multiinfarct dementia and dementia of the Alzheimer type. Arch Neurol 44:389–393, 1987

Davis KL, Hollander E, Davidson M, et al: Induction of depression with oxotremorine in patients with Alzheimer's disease. Am J Psychiatry 144:468–471, 1987

DeMuth GW, Rand BS: Atypical major depression in a patient with severe primary degenerative dementia. Am J Psychiatry 137:1609–1610, 1980

Devanand DP, Nelson JC: Concurrent depression and dementia: implications for diagnosis and treatment. J Clin Psychiatry 46:389–392, 1985

Fischer P, Simanyi M, Danielczyk W: Depression in dementia of the Alzheimer type and in multi-infarct dementia. Am J Psychiatry 147:1484–1487, 1990

Folstein MF, McHugh PR: Dementia syndrome of depression, in Alzheimer's Disease: Senile Dementia and Related Disorders (Aging, Vol 7). Edited by Katzman R, Terry RD, Bick KL. New York, Raven, 1978, pp 87–93

Greenwald BS, Kramer E: Major depression in severe dementia, in New Research Program and Abstracts: American Psychiatric Association 144th Annual Meeting, New Orleans, LA, May 11–16, 1991, p 170

Greenwald BS, Mathe AA, Mohs RC, et al: Cortisol and Alzheimer's disease, II: dexamethasone suppression, dementia severity, and affective symptoms. Am J Psychiatry 143:442–446, 1986a

Greenwald BS, Marin DB, Silverman SM: Serotoninergic treatment of screaming and banging in dementia. Lancet 2:1464–1465, 1986b

Greenwald BS, Kramer-Ginsberg E, Marin DB, et al: Dementia with coexistent major depression. Am J Psychiatry 146:1472–1478, 1989a

Greenwald BS, Kramer E, Wachter E, et al: Late life depressive pseudodementia, in New Research Program and Abstracts, American Psychiatric Association, 142nd Annual Meeting, San Francisco, CA, May 6–11, 1989b, p 97

Haupt M: Depression in Alzheimer's disease significantly improved under treatment with mianserine (letter). J Am Geriatr Soc 39:1141, 1991

Janowsky DS, Risch SC: Role of acetylcholine mechanisms in the affective disorders, in Psychopharmacology: The Third Generation of Progress. Edited by Meltzer HY. New York, Raven, 1987, pp 527–533

Jenike MA, Albert MS: The dexamethasone suppression test in patients with presenile and senile dementia of the Alzheimer's type. J Am Geriatr Soc 32:441–444, 1984

Katona CLE, Aldridge CR: The dexamethasone suppression test and depressive signs in dementia. J Affect Disord 8:83–89, 1985

Katz IR, Simpson GM, Curlik SM, et al: Pharmacologic treatment of major depression for elderly patients in residential care settings. J Clin Psychiatry 51 (7, suppl):41–47, 1990

Kaufman DM: Clinical Neurology for Psychiatrists. New York, Grune & Stratton, 1981, pp 46–47

Knesevich JW, Martin RL, Berg L, et al: Preliminary report on affective symptoms in the early stages of senile dementia of the Alzheimer type. Am J Psychiatry 140:233–235, 1983

Kraepelin E: Psychiatrie, ein Lehrbuch fur Studierende und Artzte. Leipzig, 1904. [Clinical Psychiatry: A Textbook for Students and Physicians, translated by Defendorf AR. New York, Macmillan, 1915]

Krishnan KRR, McKonald WM, Escalona PR, et al: Magnetic resonance imaging of the caudate nuclei in depression: preliminary observations. Arch Gen Psychiatry 49:553–557, 1992

LaRue A, Spar J, Hill CD: Cognitive impairment in late-life depression: clinical correlates and treatment implications. J Affect Disord 11:179–184, 1986

Lawlor BA: Serotonin and Alzheimer's disease. Psychiatric Annals 20:567–570, 1990

Lazarus LW, Newton N, Cohler B, et al: Frequency and presentation of depressive symptoms in patients with primary degenerative dementia. Am J Psychiatry 144:41–45, 1987

Lipowski ZJ: Delirium in the elderly patient. N Engl J Med 320:578–582, 1989

Lipsey JR, Robinson RG, Pearlson GD, et al: Nortriptyline treatment of post-stroke depression: a double-blind study. Lancet 1:297–300, 1984

Lipsey JR, Spencer WC, Rabins PV, et al: Phenomenological comparison of poststroke depression and functional depression. Am J Psychiatry 143:527–529, 1986

Liston EH: Clinical findings in presenile dementia: a report of 50 cases. J Nerv Ment Dis 167:337–342, 1979

Liston EH, Jarvik LF, Gerson S: Depression in Alzheimer's disease: an overview of adrenergic and cholinergic mechanisms. Compr Psychiatry 28:444–457, 1987

Lopez OL, Boller F, Becker JT, et al: Alzheimer's disease and depression: neuropsychological impairment and progression of the illness. Am J Psychiatry 147:855–860, 1990

MacKenzie TB, Robiner WN, Knopman DS: Differences between patient and family assessments of depression in Alzheimer's disease. Am J Psychiatry 146:1174–1178, 1989

Mahendra B: The dexamethasone suppression test in dementia. Am J Psychiatry 142:520–521, 1985

Mann DMA, Lincoln J, Yates PO, et al: Changes in the monoamine containing neurones of the human CNS in senile dementia. Br J Psychiatry 136:533–541, 1980

Mayberg HS, Robinson RG, Wong DF, et al: PET imaging of cortical S2 serotonin receptors after stroke: lateralized changes and relationship to depression. Am J Psychiatry 145:937–943, 1988

Mayeux R, Stern Y, Cote L, et al: Altered serotonin metabolism in depressed patients with Parkinson's disease. Neurology 34:642–646, 1984

Mayeux R, Stern Y, Williams JBW, et al: Clinical and biochemical features of depression in Parkinson's disease. Am J Psychiatry 143:756–759, 1986

McAllister TW: Overview: pseudodementia. Am J Psychiatry 140:528–533, 1983

McAllister TW, Price TRP: Severe depressive pseudodementia with and without dementia. Am J Psychiatry 139:626–629, 1982

McAllister TW, Price TRP, Ross S: Depressive syndromes in patients with brain injury, in 43rd Annual Scientific Program Abstracts, Society of Biological Psychiatry, Montreal, Canada, May 1988, p 161

Merriam AE, Aronson MK, Gaston P, et al: The psychiatric symptoms of Alzheimer's disease. J Am Geriatr Soc 36:7–12, 1988

Meyers BS, Greenberg R: Late-life delusional depression. J Affect Disord 11:133–137, 1986

Miller NE: The measurement of mood in senile brain disease: examiner ratings and self-reports, in Psychopathology in the Aged. Edited by Cole JO, Barrett JE. New York, Raven, 1980, pp 97–118

Moffatt J: The dexamethasone suppression test and dementia (letter). Am J Psychiatry 141:1019, 1984

Molchan SE, Vitiello B, Minichiello M, et al: Reciprocal changes in psychosis and mood after physostigmine in a patient with Alzheimer's disease. Arch Gen Psychiatry 48:1113–1114, 1991

Nelson JP, Rosenberg JP: ECT treatment of demented elderly patients with major depression: a retrospective study of efficacy and safety. Convulsive Therapy 7:157–163, 1991

Palmer AM, Francis PT, Benton JS, et al: Presynaptic serotonergic dysfunction in patients with Alzheimer's disease. J Neurochem 48:8–15, 1987

Parikh RM, Robinson RG: Mood and cognitive disorders following stroke, in Animal Models of Dementia: A Synaptic Neurochemical Perspective. Edited by Coyle JT. New York, Alan R Liss, 1987, pp 103–135

Parmelee PA, Katz IR, Lawton MP: Depression among institutionalized aged: assessment and prevalence estimation. J Gerontol 44:M22–M29, 1989

Pearlson GD, Ross CA, Lohr WD, et al: Association between family history of affective disorder and the depressive syndrome of Alzheimer's disease. Am J Psychiatry 147:452–456, 1990

Pearson JL, Teri L, Reifler BV, et al: Functional status and cognitive impairment in Alzheimer's patients with and without depression. J Am Geriatr Soc 37:1117–1121, 1989

Perry EK, Tomlinson BE, Blessed G, et al: Neuropathological and biochemical observations on the noradrenergic system in Alzheimer's disease. J Neurol Sci 51:279–287, 1981

Post F: Somatic and psychic factors in the treatment of elderly psychiatric patients. J Psychosom Res 10:13–19, 1966

Price TRP, McAllister TW: Safety and efficacy of ECT in depressed patients with dementia: a review of clinical experience. Convulsive Therapy 5:61–74, 1989

Procter AW, Middlemiss DN, Bowen DM: Selective loss of serotonin recognition sites in the parietal cortex in Alzheimer's disease. International Journal of Geriatric Psychiatry 3:37–44, 1988

Raskind M, Peskind E, Rivard MF, et al: Dexamethasone suppression test and cortisol circadian rhythm in primary degenerative dementia. Am J Psychiatry 139:1468–1471, 1982

Reifler BV: Arguments for abandoning the term pseudodementia. J Am Geriatr Soc 30:665–668, 1982

Reifler BV, Larson E, Hanley R: Coexistence of cognitive impairment and depression in geriatric outpatients. Am J Psychiatry 139:623–626, 1982

Reifler BV, Larson E, Teri L, et al: Dementia of the Alzheimer's type and depression. J Am Geriatr Soc 34:855–859, 1986

Reifler BV, Teri L, Raskind M, et al: Double-blind trial of imipramine in AD patients with and without depression. Am J Psychiatry 146:45–49, 1989

Reynolds CF, Kupfer DJ, Houck PR, et al: Reliable discrimination of elderly depressed and demented patients by electroencephalographic sleep data. Arch Gen Psychiatry 45:258–264, 1988

Robinson RG, Starkstein SE: Current research in affective disorders following stroke. J Neuropsychiatry Clin Neurosci 2:1–14, 1990

Roth M: The natural history of mental disorder in old age. Journal of Mental Science 101:281–301, 1955

Rovner BW, Kafonek S, Filipp L, et al: Prevalence of mental illness in a community nursing home. Am J Psychiatry 143:1446–1449, 1986

Rovner BW, Broadhead J, Spencer M, et al: Depression and Alzheimer's disease. Am J Psychiatry 146:350–353, 1989

Rovner BW, German PS, Brant LJ, et al: Depression and mortality in nursing homes. JAMA 265:993–996, 1991

Rubin EH, Kinscherf BA: Psychopathology of very mild dementia of the Alzheimer type. Am J Psychiatry 146:1017–1021, 1989

Sano M, Stern Y, Williams J, et al: Coexisting dementia and depression in Parkinson's disease. Arch Neurol 46:1284–1286, 1989

Schiffer RB, Herndon RM, Rudick RA: Treatment of pathologic laughing and weeping with amitriptyline. N Engl J Med 312:1480–1482, 1985

Shraberg D: The myth of pseudodementia: depression and the aging brain. Am J Psychiatry 135:601–603, 1978

Sim M, Sussman I: Alzheimer's disease: its natural history and differential diagnosis. J Nerv Ment Dis 135:489–499, 1962

Snow SS, Wells CE: Case studies in neuropsychiatry: diagnosis and treatment of coexistent dementia and depression. J Clin Psychiatry 42:439–441, 1981

Spar JE, Gerner R: Does the dexamethasone suppression test distinguish dementia from depression? Am J Psychiatry 139:238–240, 1982

Starkstein S, Robinson RG, Berthier ML, et al: Differential mood changes following basal ganglia vs. thalamic lesions. Arch Neurol 45:725–730, 1988

Sternberg DE, Jarvik ME: Memory functions in depression. Arch Gen Psychiatry 33:219–224, 1976

Sultzer DL, Levin HS, Mahler ME, et al: Assessment of cognitive, psychiatric, and behavioral disturbances in patients with dementia: the Neurobehavioral Rating Scale. J Am Geriatr Soc 40:549–555, 1992

Sunderland T, Lawlor BA, Molchan SE, et al: Depressive syndromes in the elderly: special concerns. Psychopharm Bull 24:567–576, 1988a

Sunderland T, Alterman IS, Yount D, et al: A new scale for the assessment of depressed mood in demented patients. Am J Psychiatry 145:955–959, 1988b

Teeter RB, Garetz FK, Miller WR, et al: Psychiatric disturbances of aged patients in skilled nursing homes. Am J Psychiatry 133:1430–1434, 1976

Tomlinson BE, Irving D, Blessed G: Cell loss in the locus coeruleus in senile dementia of Alzheimer type. J Neurol Sci 49:419–428, 1981

Truax P, Teri L: Are caregiver depression ratings of demented patients biased by their own mood? (abstract) Gerontologist 30 (Special Issue, October), 236A, 1990

Wamboldt MZ, Kalin NH, Weiler SJ: Consistent reversal of abnormal DSTs after different antidepressant therapies in a patient with dementia. Am J Psychiatry 142:100–103, 1985

Whitehouse PJ, Unnerstall JR: Neurochemistry of dementia (abstract). Alzheimer Dis Assoc Disord 2:159, 1988

Wragg RE, Jeste DV: Overview of depression and psychosis in Alzheimer's disease. Am J Psychiatry 146:577–587, 1989

Yamamoto T, Hirano A: Nucleus raphe dorsalis in Alzheimer's disease: neurofibrillary tangles and loss of large neurons. Ann Neurol 17:573–577, 1985

Yates CM, Ritchie IM, Simpson J, et al: Noradrenaline in Alzheimer-type dementia and Down Syndrome. Lancet 2:39–40, 1981

Zubenko GS, Moossy J: Major depression in primary dementia: clinical and neuropathologic correlates. Arch Neurol 45:1182–1186, 1988

Zubenko GS, Moossy J, Kopp U: Neurochemical correlates of major depression in primary dementia. Arch Neurol 47:209–214, 1990

Zweig RM, Ross CA, Hedreen JC, et al: Nucleus raphe dorsalis: the neuropathology of aminergic nuclei in Alzheimer's disease. Ann Neurol 24:233–242, 1988

Psychosis

Susan E. Molchan, M.D.
John T. Little, M.D.
Marc Cantillon, M.D.
Trey Sunderland, M.D.

*T*he psychiatric symptoms associated with Alzheimer's disease can be as disturbing, or more so, than the characteristic memory impairment of this illness—to patient and caregiver alike. These symptoms are often a primary reason for institutionalization (Steele et al. 1990). In this chapter, we focus on the variety of psychotic symptoms that occur in patients with Alzheimer's disease; the relationship of these symptoms to other clinical variables; and how the symptoms may relate to the biology of the illness, which may provide insights into mechanisms of psychosis in other disorders. Fortunately, these symptoms are an aspect of Alzheimer's disease that can be successfully treated with behavioral and pharmacological interventions (Wragg and Jeste 1988; Schneider et al. 1990).

Psychotic symptoms were described in the initial case report by Alzheimer (1907/1987), in which the patient had persecutory delusions and delusional jealousy. Since then, psychotic symptoms have been estimated to occur in 15%–75% of patients with Alzheimer's disease (Table 3–1). Most studies indicate that they occur in about 25% of patients with mild dementia and about 50% of those with more severe Alzheimer's disease (Rubin et al. 1988). Differences in prevalence rates among the various studies

Table 3–1. Studies of psychotic symptoms in patients with Alzheimer's disease

Study	N	Data source	Delusions (%)[a]	Hallucinations (%)[b]	Misidentifications	Unspecified or other psychotic symptoms (%)[c]
Rothschild 1941	31	Charts, state psychiatric hospital	23			
Liston 1978	46	Charts, general hospital psychiatric ward				32
Ballinger et al. 1982	77	Patients, general hospital geropsychiatry ward	38	34		
Berrios and Brook 1984	72	Patients, geropsychiatry referrals				26
Berrios 1985	74	Patients, geropsychiatry referrals		28		35
Berrios and Brook 1985	68	Patients, geropsychiatry referrals				34
Cummings 1985	27	Patients, neurobehavioral referrals	15			
Mayeux et al. 1985	121	Charts, patients, general hospital neurology service				38
Cummings et al. 1987	30	Patients, neurobehavioral referrals	30	3	6	
Reisberg et al. 1987	57	Charts, outpatients, AD Research Center	40	14 (vh = 7)	5	19

Study	N	Source/Setting				
Merriam et al. 1988	175	Patients, caregivers, neurology clinic	56	28	17	
Teri et al. 1988	127	Patients, geriatric clinic (prospective)	24	21		
Rubin et al. 1988	110	Outpatients, AD research center	31	vh = 15 ah = 10	23	4
Drewits and Rubin 1989	67 (1) 51 (2) 44 (3)	Outpatients, AD research center (longitudinal)	21 43 25	13 27 25	12 24 25	
Burns et al. 1990 a,b	178	Inpatients/outpatients, two psychiatric hospitals	16	17 (vh = 13, ah = 10)	30	
Chen et al. 1991	72	Patients, psychiatric hospitals, AD research center				25–47
Deutsch et al. 1991	170	Charts, AD research center	31	23.5 (vh = 20, ah = 10.5)	16	28
Forstl et al. 1991	128	Patients, geropsychiatry service (prospective)		vh = 10 ah = 8.5	31	
Lopez et al. 1991	113	Charts, AD research center	10.5	11.5 (vh = 8, ah = 3.5)	31	

(continued)

Table 3–1. Studies of psychotic symptoms in patients with Alzheimer's disease *(continued)*

Study	N	Data source	Delusions (%)[a]	Hallucinations (%)[b]	Misidentifications	Unspecified or other psychotic symptoms (%)[c]
Rosen and Zubenko 1991	32	Patients, longitudinal, geriatric service	73	67 (vh = 22, ah = 15.5)		
Zubenko et al. 1991	27	Patients, longitudinal, geriatric service				48
Jeste et al. 1992	107	Patients, AD research center	35	17 (vh = 12, ah = 6.5)		
Mendez et al. 1992	217	Charts, outpatient AD clinic			24	
Devanand et al. 1992	91	Outpatients, memory disorders clinic	18.7[d]	5.5 (vh = 4.4, ah = 1.1)	12.1[d]	4.4

Note. Empty cells represent parameters not measured in that study. All studies had 25 subjects or more. In the study by Drevets and Rubin (1989), in the *N* column, numbers in parentheses refer to severity ratings on the Clinical Dementia Rating (Hughes et al. 1982).

[a] Includes paranoid and generalized delusions; other types, including systematized, are listed in the Unspecified or Other column.
[b] vh = visual hallucinations. ah = auditory hallucinations.
[c] Includes systematized delusions and olfactory and tactile hallucinations.
[d] Further questioning decreased symptom incidence, depending on symptom definition.

probably reflect the variable diagnostic and histopathologic criteria for Alzheimer's disease used over the years, as well as different methods of determining symptoms. How symptoms are defined can also add to variability: what are called delusions in one study may be considered persecutory ideas in others. Study designs too may contribute to disparate results: epidemiological catchment-area studies, for example, may survey a very different sample from those in studies of subjects who were consecutive referrals to a dementia service. As Wragg and Jeste (1989) noted in their review of 21 studies of psychotic symptoms in Alzheimer's disease patients, isolated symptoms were more common than diagnosable psychotic disorders. Symptoms occurring with the greatest frequency in Alzheimer's disease patients are delusions, hallucinations, and misidentification syndromes (Drevets and Rubin 1989; Rosen and Zubenko 1991; Rubin et al. 1988; Wragg and Jeste 1989).

Delusions, hallucinations, and misidentification syndromes also occur in other illnesses that cause dementia. Along with Alzheimer's disease, multi-infarct dementia is one of the most frequent types of dementia. The prevalence and nature of psychotic symptoms, at least delusions and hallucinations, have been generally found to be similar or somewhat lower in Alzheimer's disease patients than in patients with multi-infarct dementia (Berrios and Brook 1985; Cummings et al. 1987; Swearer et al. 1988).

Evaluating Psychotic Symptoms

In evaluating psychotic symptoms in patients with Alzheimer's disease, it is important to determine whether unusual speech or behavior may be secondary to other factors, such as confusion or cognitive impairment (Lopez et al. 1991). A patient with little insight into the fact that he has a memory problem may, for example, misinterpret his forgetfulness and feel that someone is misplacing or stealing his belongings. Most studies describing psychotic symptoms in Alzheimer's disease patients were based on clinical diagnosis of symptoms, though a few used rating scales such as the Brief Psychiatric Rating Scale (Overall and

Gorham 1962) or others (Wragg and Jeste 1989).

The use of rating scales is helpful in documenting and following symptoms over time, in facilitating communication among clinicians about clinical findings, and in identifying symptoms or symptom clusters that may help to differentiate among various conditions causing dementia or to identify subgroups of Alzheimer's disease patients. Scales are also useful for measuring the effects of treatment (Sultzer et al. 1992). The specific instruments used to rate psychotic and other symptoms in Alzheimer's disease are described in detail in Chapter 6.

Types of Psychotic Symptoms

Delusions

Delusions—false, strongly held personal beliefs based on incorrect inferences about reality, from which a patient cannot be dissuaded—are most frequently of the paranoid type in patients with Alzheimer's disease (Burns et al. 1990a; Rubin et al. 1988; Wragg and Jeste 1989). Delusions have been reported to occur in 10%–75% of patients—with the greatest number of studies clustering in the range of estimates of 30%–38% (Table 3–1)—and to occur generally in patients with mild to moderate dementia (Rubin et al. 1988). In a few patients, delusions are a presenting symptom of the illness, as in the original patient described by Alzheimer (Alzheimer 1907/1987; Burns et al. 1990a). The most common types of delusions are of theft; patients frequently think that their money, clothes, or other belongings have been stolen (Burns et al. 1990a; Jeste et al. 1992). They will usually voice their concern and make accusations, and they may become angry and irritable. Patients may hide objects, presumably to keep them from being stolen. This behavior may foster the delusion, because they will often forget that they have hidden something, then presume it was stolen. Burns et al. (1990a) reported that in a study of 178 patients more men than women had delusions of theft; other gender differences have not been reported.

Less frequently, suspiciousness may be focused on the idea that someone is trying to harm the patient. They may think, for example, that their spouse is trying to send them to jail or that a staff member is trying to get them removed from the nursing home. Another not infrequent delusion is that of spousal infidelity (Burns et al. 1990a). Occasional patients may develop more systematized delusions (Rubin et al. 1988). Drevets and Rubin (1989) reported one patient who developed erotomania, another who believed that a new grandniece was her own baby, and another who felt that her family was coercing her to join a religious cult.

Hallucinations

From 3% to 50% of patients experience hallucinations, or false sensory perceptions (Table 3–1). In a review of 21 studies (Wragg and Jeste 1989) the median of those experiencing hallucinations was 28%. Hallucinations have been reported to occur more frequently in acute care, as compared with outpatient settings, probably reflecting dementia severity and the concurrence of other syndromes such as delirium. Hallucinations are often associated with delusions in Alzheimer's disease patients (Wragg and Jeste 1989). It has been reported that about 15%–22% are visual, 10%–13% are auditory, and 2% are olfactory (Burns et al. 1990b; Wragg and Jeste 1989). In a longitudinal study of 32 patients with autopsy-confirmed Alzheimer's disease, Rosen and Zubenko (1991) reported a higher rate for olfactory hallucinations (13%). Visual hallucinations are usually of people or animals (Burns et al. 1990; Wragg and Jeste 1989b). They range from pleasant— imagining one is seeing an old pet, for example—to frightening, as in visualizing a stranger in one's room. A number of subjects have been noted to see faces or small people in trees (Rubin et al. 1988).

Auditory hallucinations are often more vague, such as hearing "noises." Occasional reports have been made, however, of patients who have lengthy conversations with voices or command hallucinations (Burns et al. 1990b; Rubin et al. 1988). Olfactory hallucinations are even less frequent; the smell of onions and burning rubber has been reported (Rubin et al. 1988).

Misidentification Syndromes

Misidentification syndromes involve delusional systems and possibly hallucinations, as when a patient responds to perceived conversation; but they are differentiated sufficiently that they often fail to meet the definition of delusion, and they are generally discussed separately (Burns et al. 1990b; Rubin et al. 1988). The most frequently reported in the literature in general, from among a variety of psychiatric and neurological diagnoses, is Capgras' syndrome, in which the patient holds the belief that another person, usually a spouse or close relative, has been replaced by an impostor of similar appearance (Drevets and Rubin 1989; Forstl et al. 1991).

Misidentification syndromes have been described primarily in patients with schizophrenia, but there are many reports of them in patients with organic brain disease (Forstl et al. 1991; Joseph 1986; Mendez et al. 1992; Molchan et al. 1990). These syndromes have been reported to occur in 5%–31% of patients with Alzheimer's disease (Table 3–1), at various stages of the illness, and occasionally have been reported as a presenting symptom (Forstl et al. 1991). Misidentifications are distinct from prosopagnosia, a visuospatial problem in patients with bilateral occipitotemporal pathology in which faces are not visually recognized, but other features of an individual, such as voice, lead to recognition (Mendez et al. 1992).

Rubin et al. (1988) classified misidentification syndromes in Alzheimer's disease patients into three subgroups: 1) confusion concerning the presence or identity of people in the house, 2) confusion concerning the recognition of self, and 3) confusion concerning the television. Burns et al. (1990b) added a fourth category: the misidentification of people by mistaking a relative or friend for another person—for example, mistaking a spouse for a daughter or brother. Often patients with one type of misidentification syndrome display symptoms of others (Burns et al. 1990b). In a study of 110 patients with clinically diagnosed Alzheimer's disease, Rubin et al. (1988) reported that 8% imagined people in the house. They noted that patients may regard the imagined guests as friendly and may be seen conversing with them in a relaxed way or setting the table for them, or as hostile, with the patient becoming frightened and agitated. In that study 4% of the patients had a more classic Capgras' syndrome, in which they did not believe their spouses or children were who they claimed to be. Mendez et al. (1992) noted that patients with Capgras' syndrome and those with mirror-image misinterpretations were suspicious and/or paranoid and had delusions.

Concerning the recognition of self, 7% of the patients in the study by Rubin et al. (1988) could not recognize their own faces in a mirror. Again, it was noted that they may converse with the image in the mirror, as if it were a friend, or become agitated, even breaking the mirror, believing that the image is a person who is following or persecuting them. Interestingly, reaction to the mirror image may be variable in an individual patient, changing with time and mood (Molchan et al. 1990). Patients may also misidentify television images, not recognizing that people on television are merely images. One woman was described, for example, who felt that the people on television were watching her undress, so she would leave the room to change; another patient felt that he was being shot at and was frightened by the violence on the screen (Rubin et al. 1988).

In a study by Burns et al. (1990b), 30% of 178 patients with probable or possible Alzheimer's disease had a misidentification syndrome. Those with symptoms were younger, and their age at onset of the illness had been younger. Authors also found that more men than women were affected. In a prospective study by Forstl and associates (1991), 31% of 128 patients with possible or probable Alzheimer's disease exhibited symptoms of misidentification. In their sample, 25 misidentified people in their homes, 7 misidentified their own mirror images, and 7 misidentified television images as being actual people in the room. Only 2 patients exhibited symptoms consistent with Capgras' syndrome. Those with and without misidentification syndromes did not differ significantly with respect to age, age at illness onset, illness duration, or degree of cognitive impairment. Those with misidentification syndromes experienced visual hallucinations significantly more often than those without these syndromes. Using planimetric computed tomography (CT) measurements, the authors found that these patients had larger right anterior horn areas of the lateral ventricles and larger left anterior brain areas. They concluded that patients with misidentification syndromes have increased right frontal lobe degeneration relative to the left frontal lobe.

Misidentification syndromes were initially thought to be purely functional. Many cases have now been described in which there is bifrontal damage to the brain, with additional injury in the right cerebral hemisphere, especially the temporal lobe (Drevets and Rubin 1989; Forstl et al. 1991; Molchan et al. 1990). In Alzheimer's disease, neuropathological changes commonly occur in the frontal and temporal cortices (Katzman 1986). A mechanism hypothesized as an etiology for the misidentifications was the disconnection of the memory and affective functions in the limbic system and temporal lobes from the interpretive and judgmental functions of the frontal lobes (Joseph 1986). Burns et al. (1990b) speculated that the association they found between younger age and misidentification symptoms may be secondary to the greater parietal lobe involvement reported in younger patients with Alzheimer's disease.

Psychosis and the Course and Severity of Dementia

In relating the occurrence of psychotic symptoms to clinical stage or severity of the illness, findings from studies differ (Wragg and Jeste 1989). Results from a number of studies have suggested that patients with delusions have moderate levels of dementia (Berrios and Brook 1985; Drevets and Rubin 1989; Rubin et al. 1988). Cummings (1985) hypothesized that some cognitive integrity is needed for delusions to occur and be maintained. Still others found that those with psychosis, especially hallucinations, were more cognitively impaired than those without it (Merriam et al. 1988; Rosen and Zubenko 1991; Wragg and Jeste 1989), although psychotic symptoms have been reported to be rare in patients with very severe dementia (Burns et al. 1990b; Jeste et al. 1992). As Jeste et al. suggested, this may be a reflection of the deterioration in verbal abilities in these patients. Consistent with an earlier study by Stern et al. (1987), Drevits and Rubin (1989) concluded that psychotic symptoms are associated with a faster rate of cognitive decline in Alzheimer's disease, although not with increased mortality. Their conclusions were based on results from a longitudinal study in which many of the subjects' diagnoses were confirmed at autopsy. After 66 months of follow-up, those with psychotic symptoms had a 20% mortality rate, as opposed to 60% for those without psychosis. Burns et al. (1990a) did not find a relationship between the presence of delusions and the rate of decline, although they did find that those with hallucinations had deteriorated to a greater degree at 12-month follow-up than those without hallucinations (Burns et al. 1990b). Those authors also found that patients with misidentification syndromes had a significantly decreased 30-month mortality rate.

In a longitudinal study, Rosen and Zubenko (1991) found that rates of psychosis increased with increasing dementia severity; half of the patients with scores of less than 10 on the Mini-Mental State Exam had psychotic symptoms. Rosen and Zubenko found that psychosis was associated with more rapid cognitive decline but not with increased mortality. They also reported that once psychotic symptoms were present, they remitted without treatment in only 13% of patients. Why psychotic symptoms are associated with more rapid cognitive decline is unknown. As Rosen and Zubenko speculated, the pathology that causes psychotic symptoms may be particularly virulent, or the presence of psychotic symptoms may interfere with performance on cognitive tests. Or, as speculated by Burns et al. (1990b) and others, those with psychotic symptoms may receive different patterns of care than those without them. More longitudinal and prospective studies on the relationship between psychotic symptoms and cognitive decline are needed.

Psychosis and Neuropsychological Impairment

Few studies have examined patterns of neuropsychological impairment in relation to psychotic symptoms. Jeste et al. (1992) reported that 37 patients with delusions performed significantly worse on a test of memory, on two tests designed to evaluate frontal lobe function, and on a test of category fluency (a measure of retrieval from knowledge memory) than did 70 patients without delusions. They interpreted the poorer performance of delusional patients on these tasks as reflecting greater frontal and temporal dysfunction.

Lopez et al. (1991) found that patients with psychosis had a defect in receptive language, as measured by tests of auditory and reading comprehension. Interestingly, as those authors noted, patients with Wernicke's aphasia, who also have comprehension deficits, have been reported to experience psychotic episodes. They also noted that there were no differences in the neuropsychological profiles of patients with and without visual hallucinations, indicating that impairment in visual information processing, mediated by the occipitoparietal cortex, cannot explain these symptoms in Alzheimer's disease. They also found that psychotic patients were more likely to have abnormal EEGs, with increased delta and theta activity, which they interpreted as an indication of a greater degree of cerebral dysfunction. There was no difference in the pattern of abnormalities (focal or generalized) between those with and those without psychosis, or in right-left predominance of abnormalities.

Other Clinical Symptoms and Psychosis

Attempts have been made to examine which clinical symptoms may predispose to or associate with psychotic symptoms in Alzheimer's disease. Sensory impairment, for example, was found to be more common in elderly patients with psychosis, with or without dementia. In Alzheimer's disease, however, sensory impairment has not been associated with psychosis, although few studies have examined this association (Wragg and Jeste 1989).

The age at onset of symptoms of Alzheimer's disease may be a characteristic of illness subgroups. No difference in the presence of psychotic symptoms has been reported between patients who had an early age at onset and those who had a late one (Drevets and Rubin 1989), although few studies have examined this association.

The presence of psychosis may help to distinguish between clinical and neuropathological subtypes of this heterogeneous illness. Alzheimer's disease patients with extrapyramidal symptoms were reported to have psychotic symptoms almost twice as frequently as those without extrapyramidal symptoms, to be more cognitively impaired, and to have a faster rate of cognitive decline (Mayeux et al. 1985; Stern et al. 1987). Patients with myoclonus were also found to have a greater frequency of psychotic symptoms and to be more cognitively impaired than those without myoclonus (Mayeux et al. 1985). The authors speculated that these symptom constellations may reflect a more severe and generalized form of Alzheimer's disease. Chen et al. (1991), in a longitudinal study of 72 patients, found that psychotic and extrapyramidal symptoms were more likely to occur in the first few years of illness than later. They noted that the association of faster disease progression with these signs make them prognostic indicators that should help in treatment planning. They also suggested that, rather than defining subtypes of Alzheimer's disease, such symptoms may characterize the progression of the illness.

The association between psychosis and extrapyramidal symptoms was not confirmed in another longitudinal study of 32 patients (Rosen and Zubenko 1991). In this study, 22% of patients met criteria for major depression. In only two of these patients were psychotic symptoms concurrent with the depression, suggesting that psychotic and depressive syndromes may arise from different pathological substrates in many patients with this illness. This possibility is supported by data from neuropathological studies, as described below.

A number of authors have noted that patients with psychotic symptoms, most notably delusions, have more frequent episodes of violent behavior than those without psychosis. In a longitudinal study of 181 patients with moderate to severe probable Alzheimer's disease, Deutsch et al. (1991) reported that delusions and misidentification syndromes often preceded episodes of physical aggression. Of the patients in their sample, 29.6% were reported to exhibit physically aggressive behavior; other studies have reported incidences of up to 47% (Deutsch et al. 1991). Lopez and associates (1991) found that patients with psychotic symptoms were more frequently aggressive and hostile—with behaviors ranging from uncooperativeness to physical violence—than those without psychosis. Most of those with such symptoms were treated with antipsychotic medication; by the time of a follow-up visit, therefore, the rates of hostile or aggressive behaviors between those with and those without a history of psychosis did not differ.

Pathophysiological Mechanisms of Psychosis

In psychoses associated with various organic brain disorders, lesions have often been localized to subcortical (basal ganglia, thalamus, and midbrain) and limbic structures (Cummings 1985; Terry and Davies 1980). Some of these areas are characteristically sites of severe neuropathology in Alzheimer's disease, such as the hippocampus, amygdala, temporal cortex, and frontal cortex (Katzman 1986). Also, as in Alzheimer's disease (Haxby et al. 1988), patients with psychoses presenting earlier in life have been shown to have decreased blood flow (Weinberger et al. 1986; Zubenko 1992) and glucose metabolism (Buchsbaum et al. 1984; Zubenko 1992) in the frontal cortex.

In a study of 27 patients with autopsy-confirmed Alzheimer's disease by Zubenko et al. (1991), those with a history of psychosis had increased numbers of cortical senile plaques and neurofibrillary tangles, especially in the prosubiculum and middle frontal cortex, respectively, compared with those who had not had psychotic symptoms. The authors speculated that the larger numbers of these characteristic lesions of Alzheimer's disease may be related to the increased rates of cognitive decline in the psychotic subgroup. They also noted that these degenerative changes may be part of the reason why psychotic symptoms in Alzheimer's disease patients are persistent and why the symptoms may be more resistant to pharmacological treatment. Patients with psychosis also had relative preservation of norepinephrine in the substantia nigra, with trends toward preservation in other brain regions, indicating, as the authors speculated, that for psychotic symptoms to occur, some minimum degree of noradrenergic functioning may be necessary. Levels of serotonin were decreased in the prosubiculum of the hippocampus, with trends toward reductions in other cortical and subcortical regions. Notably, the pattern of neurochemical changes is different from that reported in Alzheimer's disease with major depression, which included degeneration in the locus coeruleus and substantia nigra.

As Cummings (1985) hypothesized from data on anatomical sites of pathology across a variety of organic brain disorders, delusions appear to arise from the disruption of connections between limbic and cortical areas. Disruption of limbic-subcortical systems that mediate mood, motivation, and assignment of emotional significance to experiences may result in abnormal emotional experiences, which, as interpreted and elaborated by hemispheric cortical regions, result in delusions. Dopaminergic pathways may be affected by lesions in the limbic or subcortical regions; this is hypothesized to occur in schizophrenic patients, in whom delusions are predominant symptoms. Lesions may also affect cortical regions and contribute to the occurrence of delusions. Right temporoparietal lesions, for example, may result in abnormal perceptual input to the limbic system (Cummings 1985).

The brain areas most affected by senile plaques and neurofibrillary tangles in Alzheimer's disease patients are in the limbic system (hippocampus, amygdala, and temporal lobe) as well as the frontal cortex (Katzman 1986; Terry and Davies 1980). Neuropathological changes in the limbic system have also been identified in another neuropsychiatric disease, schizophrenia, in which psychotic symptoms are characteristic (Brown et al. 1986; Conrad et al. 1991). Symptoms in both illnesses often respond to treatment with neuroleptic medication. For many years, the primary theory of the mechanism of action of neuroleptics has been their ability to block mesocorticolimbic dopamine receptors. Elaborations on this theory, including the contribution of other neurotransmitter systems to the production and amelioration of psychotic symptoms, have been promoted in the last few years. One that may have some relevance to such symptoms in Alzheimer's disease patients, who have well-documented severe deficits in the cholinergic system, has been discussed by Tandon and Greden (1989) in reference to schizophrenia and involves cholinergic-dopaminergic interactions. The authors reviewed evidence that decreased cholinergic activity relative to dopaminergic activity may be associated with psychotic symptoms, and the inverse with negative and depressive symptoms. In Alzheimer's disease patients, the loss of cholinergic system activity may allow a disinhibition of the dopaminergic system and contribute to the production of delusions and hallucinations. Besides the response of these symptoms to neuroleptic medication, further support for this idea is illustrated in a report of a patient with moderately severe Alzheimer's disease, in which a very clear association was demonstrated between the alleviation of delusions and hallucinations and treatment with the cholinesterase inhibitor physostigmine. A decrease in the cerebrospinal fluid level of the dopamine metabolite homovanillic acid was shown to occur concurrent with this decrease in psychotic symptoms (Molchan et al. 1991). Such observations are an indication that some symptoms in various neuropsychiatric disorders may have overlapping structural and neurochemical substrates.

Conclusions

Further clinical characterization of psychotic symptoms in Alzheimer's disease patients is needed, through case and large cross-sectional studies as well as prospective, longitudinal studies. In addition, the biological substrates of psychotic symptoms in Alzheimer's disease can be explored with the same tools used to explore these symptoms in other illnesses, such as sleep studies and neuroendocrine and pharmacological probes. Brain-imaging techniques such as positron-emission tomography (PET) and single photon emission computed tomography (SPECT) should also contribute to neuroanatomical and neurophysiological data on these questions. More postmortem neurochemical and neuropathological studies are needed. Careful studies of which treatments are helpful for which specific symptoms can also provide information on, for example, which neurotransmitter systems may be involved in psychosis in patients with dementia. This information may be valuable in providing clues to the pathophysiology of other psychiatric disorders. Furthermore, because there is currently no treatment for the cognitive abnormalities associated with Alzheimer's disease, the psychiatric symptoms stand out as potentially remediable with clinically available medications. The refinement of treatments for psychotic symptoms should delay nursing home placement for more individuals and would alleviate some of the burdens associated with Alzheimer's disease for patients and caregivers alike.

References

Alzheimer A: Uber eigenartige erkrankung der hirnrinde. Cbl Nervenheilk Psychiatrie 18:177–179, 1907. [About a peculiar disease of the cerebral cortex, translated by Jarvik L, Greenson H. Alzheimer Dis Assoc Disord 1:7–8, 1987]

Ballinger BR, Reid AH, Heather BB: Cluster analysis of symptoms in elderly demented patients. Br J Psychiatry 140:257–262, 1982

Berrios GE: Presbyophrenia: clinical aspects. Br J Psychiatry 147:76–79, 1985

Berrios GE, Brook P: Visual hallucinations and sensory delusions in the elderly. Br J Psychiatry 144:662–664, 1984

Berrios GE, Brook P: Delusions and the psychopathology of the elderly with dementia. Acta Psychiatr Scand 72:296–301, 1985

Brown R, Colter N, Corsellis JAN, et al: Postmortem evidence of structural brain changes in schizophrenia. Arch Gen Psychiatry 43:36–42, 1986

Buchsbaum MS, Delisi LE, Holocomb HH, et al: Anteroposterior gradients in cerebral glucose use in schizophrenia and affective disorders. Arch Gen Psychiatry 41:1159–1166, 1984

Burns A, Jacoby R, Levy R: Psychiatric phenomena in Alzheimer's disease, I: disorders of thought content. Br J Psychiatry 157:72–76, 1990a

Burns A, Jacoby R, Levy R: Psychiatric phenomena in Alzheimer's disease, II: disorders of perception. Br J Psychiatry 157:76–81, 1990b

Chen JY, Stern Y, Sano M, et al: Cumulative risks of developing extrapyramidal signs, psychosis, or myoclonus in the course of Alzheimer's disease. Arch Neurol 48:1141–1143, 1991

Conrad AJ, Abebe T, Austin R, et al: Hippocampal pyramidal cell disarray in schizophrenia as a bilateral phenomenon. Arch Gen Psychiatry 48:413–417, 1991

Cummings JL: Organic delusions: phenomenology, anatomical correlations, and review. Br J Psychiatry 146:184–197, 1985

Cummings JL, Miller B, Hill MA, et al: Neuropsychiatric aspects of multi-infarct dementia and dementia of the Alzheimer type. Arch Neurol 44:389–393, 1987

Deutsch LH, Bylsma FW, Rovner BW, et al: Psychosis and physical aggression in probable Alzheimer's disease. Am J Psychiatry 148:1159–1163, 1991

Devanand DP, Miller L, Richard SM, et al: The Columbia University Scale for psychopathology in Alzheimer's Disease. Arch Neurol 49:371–376, 1992

Drevets WC, Rubin EH: Psychotic symptoms and the longitudinal course of senile dementia of the Alzheimer type. Biol Psychiatry 25:39–48, 1989

Forstl H, Burns A, Jacoby R, et al: Neuroanatomical correlates of clinical misidentification and misperception in senile dementia of the Alzheimer type. J Clin Psychiatry 52:268–271, 1991

Haxby JV, Grady CL, Koss E, et al: Heterogeneous anterior-posterior metabolic patterns in dementia of the Alzheimer type. Neurology 38:1853–1863, 1988

Hughes CP, Berg L, Danziger WL, et al: A new clinical scale for the staging of dementia. Br J Psychiatry 140:566–572, 1982

Jeste DV, Wragg RE, Salmon DP, et al: Cognitive deficits of patients with Alzheimer's disease with and without delusions. Am J Psychiatry 149:184–189, 1992

Joseph AB: Focal central nervous system abnormalities in patients with misidentification syndromes. Bibliotheca Psychiatrica (Basel) 164:68–79, 1986

Katzman R: Medical progress: Alzheimer's disease. N Engl J Med 314:964–972, 1986

Lopez OL, Becker JT, Brenner RP, et al: Alzheimer's disease with delusions and hallucinations: neuropsychological and electroencephalographic correlates. Neurology 41:906–912, 1991

Mayeux R, Stern Y, Spanton S: Heterogeneity in dementia of the Alzheimer type: evidence of subgroups. Neurology 35:453–461, 1985

Mendez MF, Martin RJ, Smyth KA, et al: Disturbances of person identification in Alzheimer's disease. J Nerv Ment Dis 180:94–96, 1992

Merriam AE, Aronson MK, Gaston P, et al: The psychiatric symptoms of Alzheimer's disease. J Am Geriatr Soc 36:7–12, 1988

Molchan SE, Martinez RA, Lawlor BA, et al: Reflections of the self: atypical misidentification and delusional syndromes in two patients with Alzheimer's disease. Br J Psychiatry 157:605–608, 1990

Molchan SE, Vitiello B, Minichiello M, et al: Reciprocal changes in psychosis and mood after physostigmine in a patient with Alzheimer's disease (letter). Arch Gen Psychiatry 48:1113, 1991

Overall JE, Gorham DR: The Brief Psychiatric Rating Scale. Psychol Rep 10:799–812, 1962

Reisberg B, Borenstein J, Salob SP, et al: Behavioral symptoms in Alzheimer's disease: phenomenologoy and treatment. J Clin Psychiatry 48:9–15, 1987

Rosen J, Zubenko GS: Emergence of psychosis and depression in the longitudinal evaluation of Alzheimer's disease. Biol Psychiatry 29:224–232, 1991

Rothschild D: The clinical differentiation of senile and arteriosclerotic psychoses. Am J Psychiatry 98:324–333, 1941

Rubin EH, Drevets WC, Burke WJ: The nature of psychotic symptoms in senile dementia of the Alzheimer type. J Geriatr Psychiatry Neurol 1:16–20, 1988

Schneider LS, Pollock VE, Lyness SA: A metaanalysis of controlled trials of neuroleptic treatment in dementia. J Am Geriatr Soc 38:553–563, 1990

Steele C, Rovner B, Chase GA, et al: Psychiatric symptoms and nursing home placement of patients with Alzheimer's disease. Am J Psychiatry 147:1049–1051, 1990

Stern Y, Mayeux R, Sano M, et al: Predictors of disease course in patients with probable Alzheimer's disease. Neurology 37:1649–1653, 1987

Sultzer DL, Levin HS, Mahler ME, et al: Assessment of cognitive, psychiatric and behavioral disturbances in patients with dementia: the neurobehavioral rating scale. J Am Geriatr Soc 40:549–555, 1992

Swearer JM, Drachman DA, O'Donnell BF, et al: Troublesome and disruptive behaviors in dementia. J Am Geriatr Soc 36:784–790, 1988

Tandon R, Greden JF: Cholinergic hyperactivity and negative schizophrenic symptoms: a model of cholinergic/dopaminergic interactions in schizophrenia. Arch Gen Psychiatry 46:745–753, 1989

Teri L, Larson EB, Reifler BV: Behavioral disturbance in dementia of the Alzheimer's type. J Am Geriatr Soc 36:1–6, 1988

Terry RD, Davies P: Dementia of the Alzheimer type. Annu Rev Neurosci 3:77–95, 1980

Weinberger DR, Berman KF, Zec RF: Physiologic dysfunction of dorsolateral prefrontal cortex in schizophrenia. Arch Gen Psychiatry 43:114–124, 1986

Wragg RE, Jeste DV: Neuroleptics and alternative treatments: management of behavioral symptoms and psychosis in Alzheimer's disease and related conditions. Psychiatr Clin North Am 11:195–213, 1988

Wragg RE, Jeste DV: Overview of depression and psychosis in Alzheimer's disease. Am J Psychiatry 146:577–587, 1989

Zubenko GS: Biological correlates of clinical heterogeneity in primary dementia. Neuropsychopharmacology 6:77–93, 1992

Zubenko GS, Moossy J, Martinez J, et al: Neuropathologic and neurochemical correlates of psychosis in primary dementia. Arch Neurol 48:619–624, 1991

Section II

Biomedical and Quantitative Aspects of Behavioral Symptoms

CHAPTER 4

Medical Contributions to Development of Behavioral Symptoms

Paul S. Aisen, M.D.

Alzheimer's disease is a devastating, slowly but relentlessly progressive illness with protean manifestations, including not only cognitive dysfunction but behavioral and eventually physical manifestations as well. The disease itself changes very gradually. An acute change, whether it is a sudden cognitive worsening or a new behavioral problem, should suggest to the clinician that a complication, such as a toxic drug effect or a comorbid medical condition, has developed. Whereas at this time the treatment of Alzheimer's disease is empirical and symptomatic, the identification of a superimposed medical problem can lead to specific, effective measures that eliminate the cause of the deterioration, resulting in clinical improvement.

The clinician's task is complicated by several difficulties. In the geriatric population in general, atypical presentations of medical conditions are the rule. In the treatment of patients with dementia, medical diagnosis is further obscured by the patient's impaired ability to understand and communicate symptoms. In the common situation of sudden cognitive or behavioral deterioration, clues to specific diagnosis are often scarce. To minimize errors, the physician must be familiar with the wide range of potential medical complications and must maintain an open and skeptical mind.

A Broad Concept of Delirium

The term *delirium* applies to an organic brain syndrome of acute onset that may be manifested as cognitive or behavioral dysfunction. The full-blown syndrome is easy to recognize on the basis of the following DSM-IV diagnostic features (American Psychiatric Association 1994): impairment of attention, disorganized thinking with incoherent speech, reduced level of consciousness, illusions or hallucinations, disturbed sleep-wake cycle, increased or decreased psychomotor activity, disorientation, and memory impairment. Delirium usually has an acute or subacute onset, with fluctuations in clinical signs during the course of a day.

The cognitive and perceptual deficits of delirium and dementia overlap, and the distinction between these two syndromes may be difficult (Lipowski 1989; Rabins and Folstein 1982). The Mini-Mental State Exam (MMSE) (Folstein et al. 1975) is the most commonly used screening tool for delirium (Lindesay et al. 1990), but it does not differentiate delirium from dementia (Anthony et al. 1982). In the setting of Alzheimer's disease, the most useful signs of delirium are an acute change in behavior and/or cognition, with rapid fluctuations, and impairment of attention. Clinical examination is often inconclusive; history obtained from family and caregivers and observation over time are essential.

A practical definition of delirium in the setting of dementia is an acute cognitive or behavioral decline that reverses with removal of the etiological insult. Thus, in the common situation of an unexplained clinical deterioration, such as increased agitation, a presumptive diagnosis of delirium should be made, and efforts to identify potential causes should ensue. Improvement of the patient's condition following adjustment of medications or effective treatment of a medical problem retrospectively confirms the diagnosis of delirium.

Pathophysiology of Delirium

The characterization of delirium as reversible, generalized cerebral insufficiency was first proposed by Engel and Romano (1959) and has been reemphasized by Blass and colleagues (1991). Positron-emission tomography (PET) studies indicate that global cognitive dysfunction, whether a fixed dementia or reversible delirium, is associated with reduced cerebral metabolism (Phelps et al. 1982). Evidence for diffuse cortical dysfunction in delirium also includes the characteristic diffuse slowing of background activity on electroencephalography (EEG) (Engel and Romano 1959; Lipowski 1990). This pattern of EEG abnormality is much more common in delirium than in dementia of mild or moderate severity, and it may thus be useful in distinguishing between them (Rabins and Folstein 1982). Because the severity of clinical impairment in delirium correlates with the degree of abnormality of the EEG, serial EEG tracings have been advocated to monitor the response to therapy (Brenner 1991).

Many conditions can contribute to impairment of cortical neuron function and lead to delirium. Cerebral metabolism may be directly affected by hypoxia, hypoglycemia, hypothyroidism, and hypoperfusion (i.e., low cardiac output). Endogenous or exogenous toxins can cause neuronal dysfunction. Situations in which endogenous toxins are implicated include uremia, hepatic encephalopathy, and hypercalcemia. Intoxication with or withdrawal from exogenous agents, including alcohol and both illicit and prescription drugs, may also affect cerebral metabolism or neurotransmission.

The neurotransmitter most closely associated with cognitive function is acetylcholine (Drachman and Leavitt 1974). It is thus not surprising that drugs with anticholinergic effects can all too frequently cause delirium. Alzheimer's disease, and to a lesser extent aging, are associated with loss of neurons and cholinergic transmission (Perry et al. 1992); this presumably contributes to the increased risk of delirium in elderly people and in patients with Alzheimer's disease.

It is likely that multiple neurotransmitters play a role in delirium. The cortical arousal system involves the interaction of cholinergic, serotonergic, and noradrenergic systems (Hobson et al. 1986), each of which has therefore been implicated in the pathophysiology of delirium (Lindesay et al. 1990; Lipowski 1990). Other putative factors include cortisol (Kral 1975), glutamate and gamma-aminobutyric acid (Lipowski 1990), and beta-endorphins (Koponen et al. 1989).

Medical Illness and Delirium

In the setting of significant brain disease such as Alzheimer's disease, delirium can accompany seemingly minor insults. Among the most common examples of this is the urinary tract infection. In one study, 26% of patients admitted to a psychogeriatric unit over a 2-year period with a diagnosis of delirium had urinary tract infections (Manepalli et al. 1990). Of these patients, 71% had underlying dementia. Although in the majority of cases the urinary tract infections were asymptomatic and not associated with systemic signs of infection, in 64% the delirium cleared with appropriate antibiotic treatment. Although there are many possible confounding factors (such as acclimation to environmental change) in this type of study, the conclusion is justified that urinary tract infection is an important treatable cause of delirium in elderly patients with dementia. Many infectious-disease specialists advise against the treatment of "asymptomatic" urinary tract infections in elderly, institutionalized patients. However, in a patient with dementia and recent behavioral deterioration, treatment of pyuria is indicated.

The mechanism by which an apparently asymptomatic urinary tract infection can precipitate delirium in a susceptible patient is not clear. Possibly the infection causes discomfort that the patient is not able to communicate. Clinical experience indicates that any physical discomfort can cause behavioral or cognitive worsening. A common example is fecal impaction; changes in bowel habits must be monitored, investigated when appropriate, and treated.

The insult that precipitates clinical deterioration need not be physical. A change in sensory stimulation may result in agitation, confusion, hallucinations, and delusions. "Sundowning," or transient nocturnal confusion in institutionalized elderly patients (Evans 1987), is an example of delirium in the broad sense. Progression of hearing or visual deficits may contribute to behavioral problems; evaluation and treatment of such deficits may be clinically rewarding. The relatively common occurrence of delirium following eye surgery has been attributed to sensory deprivation, although other factors such as dehydration and the perioperative use of sedatives and anticholinergic eye drops may be important (Burrows et al. 1985; Karhunen and Raitta 1982).

In the patient with dementia, major medical illnesses may present as delirium, with few clues to the correct specific diagnosis. Such diverse conditions as myocardial ischemia, cholecystitis, and gastrointestinal cancer may present with a similar clinical picture in the setting of Alzheimer's disease. Any clinical change must be approached with a thorough medical evaluation. Fecal impaction, decubitus ulcer, and cellulitis are examples of common remediable medical conditions readily diagnosed by routine physical examination. Hyponatremia, hypercalcemia, hypothyroidism, and pernicious anemia are conditions easily diagnosed with routine laboratory tests. The extent to which a specific diagnosis is pursued must be tempered by the likelihood that correct diagnosis will lead to effective therapy. Thus an invasive workup to document suspected pancreatic cancer may not be appropriate.

Drugs and Delirium

Polypharmacy is a major issue in geriatric medicine, of paramount importance to clinicians treating patients with Alzheimer's disease. A great deal of harm is done inadvertently to these patients by the casual prescription of medications. Patients and their families identify many complaints and ailments; agitation, insomnia, constipation, and musculoskeletal pain are a few of the most common. These complaints are real and important; as noted above, even minor discomforts can lead to general deterioration in an Alzheimer's disease patient. But the most facile remedy, writing a prescription, frequently does more harm than good.

Several factors contribute to the very high rate of drug toxicity in this population (Lipowski 1989). Cognitive and sensory deficits increase the likelihood of errors in understanding and following instructions regarding medication use. The common practice of consulting multiple physicians can lead to multiple prescriptions without adequate consideration of potential adverse drug interactions. Therapeutic dosages of many drugs are difficult to predict for elderly patients. Variations in the absorption, distribution, receptor binding, metabolism, and elimination of drugs among elderly patients lead to the unpredictability of responses.

Psychotropic Drugs

Psychotropic drugs are among the most likely to cause cognitive or behavioral toxicity. Medications with anticholinergic properties are the classic examples of delirium-inducing drugs. This fact should be an important consideration in deciding among psychotropics. When a tricyclic antidepressant is indicated for the treatment of depression in a patient with Alzheimer's disease, secondary amines such as nortriptyline and desipramine are less anticholinergic and therefore preferable to tertiary amines such as amitriptyline and imipramine (Davidson 1992; Jarvik 1981).

Choosing among neuroleptic drugs is more complicated. Haloperidol and similar high-potency neuroleptics are often selected to treat psychotic symptoms in patients with dementia. The high-potency neuroleptics have the least anticholinergic potential, causing less cognitive impairment, sedation, and hypotension than lower-potency drugs (Jenike 1989). Haloperidol, however, may cause extrapyramidal toxicity at very low doses in elderly patients with dementia. If it is necessary to add an anticholinergic or dopaminergic drug to a high-potency neuroleptic to treat secondary parkinsonism, the risk of delirium becomes high. Some clinicians use low-potency neuroleptics despite the greater anticholinergic effects, particularly when some sedation is desired or to avoid extrapyramidal toxicity. When any neuroleptic drug is prescribed to a patient with Alzheimer's disease, regular quantitative assessment of the behavioral and cognitive effects are important.

Sedative drugs such as the benzodiazepines are commonly prescribed for sleep disorders in patients with dementia. Elderly patients are particularly sensitive to these drugs (Meyer 1982); toxic effects include oversedation, increased risk of falls (Sorock and Shimkin 1988; Tinetti et al. 1988), cognitive worsening, and frank delirium (Tune and Bylsma 1991). The pharmacological effect of benzodiazepines may be very long: diazepam has a mean half-life of 79 hours in patients over age 60 (Salzman et al. 1983). To minimize the risk of prolonged toxic reactions, short-acting benzodiazepines such as lorazepam should be used.

Some clinicians prefer to prescribe chloral hydrate rather than benzodiazepines when a sedative is indicated for patients with dementia. Chloral hydrate may have a lower potential for dependency, and it has not been documented to increase the risk of falls. However, chloral hydrate has been reported to cause delirium in patients with Alzheimer's disease (Tune and Bylsma 1991).

Nonpsychiatric Drugs

Drugs prescribed for nonpsychiatric indications are most likely to produce behavioral symptoms or delirium when they have central nervous system (CNS) activity or significant anticholinergic effects. Examples of the former include propranolol, a beta-adrenergic receptor blocker with CNS activity used to treat hypertension (Husserl and Messerli 1981), angina, and arrhythmias; and methyldopa, a central adrenergic receptor agonist prescribed for hypertension (Adler 1974). Other drugs repeatedly linked to delirium include the histamine H_2 receptor blocker cimetidine; the antiparkinsonian agents levodopa, bromocriptine, and amantadine; digoxin; corticosteroids; nonsteroidal anti-inflammatory drugs; and narcotic analgesics (Lipowski 1990). The Medical Letter (1989) lists hundreds of nonpsychiatric drugs that may cause delirium. Recent studies employing a radioreceptor assay suggest that many commonly used drugs may have previously underestimated anticholinergic effects, accounting for their capacity to induce delirium; examples include isosorbide, ranitidine, and nifedipine (Tune and Bylsma 1991).

Over-the-counter medications may cause delirium in susceptible individuals. For example, diphenhydramine, an over-the-
counter antihistamine, has significant anticholinergic properties.
Many people do not consider products available over the counter
to be "medications," and they therefore do not report their use to
physicians. Patients and families may also neglect to report the
use of eye drops, which may in fact have systemic anticholinergic
effects that contribute to delirium (Lipowski 1990).

Although there is great variability in the potential of medications to cause behavioral and cognitive toxicity, it is wise to
assume when treating patients who have Alzheimer's disease
that any drug with systemic effects can cause delirium. In other
words, in evaluating a patient with a recent deterioration, sus-
pect any medication to which the patient has been exposed.
Wherever feasible, medications should be tapered or discontinued. When a medication is considered essential, substitution of
alternatives with less potential to cause delirium should be considered. For example, a patient requiring beta-blocker therapy for
angina could be switched from propranolol to the less CNS-
active agent atenolol.

Susceptibility to delirium should be considered before drugs
are prescribed to patients with Alzheimer's disease. The threshold for the treatment of hypertension should be higher than in
patients without brain disease; the risk of delirium and other
adverse effects of treatment may outweigh the reduction in cerebrovascular events. In particular, as noted above, medications to
be avoided are centrally active beta-adrenergic receptor blockers,
such as propranolol (Husserl and Messerli 1981), and alpha-
adrenergic receptor agonists, such as methyldopa (Adler 1974)
and clonidine (Houston 1981). The benefit of digoxin in the treatment of compensated heart failure may not justify the high incidence of delirium with this medication (Bigger 1985). Other
common examples in which the risk of drug toxicity usually
outweighs the benefit in Alzheimer's disease include the use of
theophylline to treat chronic obstructive lung disease, nonsteroidal anti-inflammatory agents for osteoarthritis, narcotic analgesics for any chronic condition, antiarrhythmic drugs for
asymptomatic ventricular ectopy, and histamine H_2 receptor an-
tagonists for dyspepsia.

Treatment of Delirium

The critical issues in the management of delirium in patients with Alzheimer's disease are recognition of the syndrome and minimization of any potential contributing factors. Delirium must be suspected in any patient with an acute or subacute decline. The first steps should therefore be a comprehensive history (usually consisting primarily of interviews with family members and caregivers) and a physical examination, with particular attention to drug exposure and the identification of physical and medical disorders. The routine workup should include urinalysis, complete blood count, electrolytes, urea nitrogen and creatinine, calcium, liver chemistries, B_{12} level, thyroid function tests (including thyrotropin), chest X ray, and electrocardiogram. The results of these studies may lead to further investigation, but the clinician must always weigh the expense, discomfort, and risk of each procedure against the likelihood of uncovering a treatable condition. Patients with dementia who are agitated may require sedation before some procedures (e.g., magnetic resonance imaging [MRI]), and the necessary sedation may carry the risk of aspiration.

EEG may be useful under certain circumstances. If the underlying dementia is mild and therefore not likely to be associated with EEG abnormalities, diffuse background slowing on EEG supports a diagnosis of delirium. Improvement in the EEG may be a guide to clinical response to treatment measures (Brenner 1991).

In most cases, observation and supportive care are appropriate while the patient's response to interventions (i.e., adjustment of medications and treatment of medical conditions) is followed. Particular attention must be paid to maintaining adequate fluid and electrolyte balance. Attentive nursing care, with frequent reassurance and reorientation, will minimize agitation and the need for pharmacological or physical restraints. Recovery may be slow; even when delirium is precipitated by a drug with rapid clearance, it may take a week after discontinuation before significant clinical improvement occurs.

Haloperidol is the drug most often recommended for the management of delirium, because it is effective in treating delusions, hallucinations, and agitation and it does not often cause hypotension or cardiovascular toxicity (Lipowski 1990). However, in Alzheimer's disease with superimposed delirium, the risks of this treatment usually outweigh the benefits. These patients are at very high risk for extrapyramidal toxicity, and the coadministration of an anticholinergic drug is virtually contraindicated. Haloperidol itself has anticholinergic properties (albeit less than other neuroleptics); on this basis, it may cause delirium or may exacerbate delirium induced by the anticholinergic effects of other drugs. This again underlines the importance of making a careful evaluation before treating behavioral complications in Alzheimer's disease. Unless mandated by severe agitation, no psychotropic drugs should be administered to the patient with dementia who possibly has delirium.

In the unusual case of florid drug-induced anticholinergic delirium, with evidence of muscarinic blockade such as tachycardia, hypertension, dilated pupils, facial flushing, and constipation, specific treatment with physostigmine may be considered (Lipowski 1990). Physostigmine is a short-acting anticholinesterase with CNS activity. It can be administered in intramuscular or intravenous doses of 1–2 mg every 2 hours. The most common side effect of physostigmine is nausea, but bronchospasm and bradycardia can occur.

There are a few reports of the successful treatment of delirium with electroconvulsive therapy (Kramp and Bolwig 1981; Roberts 1963). This modality should be reserved for the rare delirious patient with severe agitation and/or psychosis who does not respond to or does not tolerate haloperidol and benzodiazepines.

Avoiding Delirium: Principles of Optimal Medical Care

Prevention would be far preferable to even optimal recognition and treatment of delirium. Unfortunately, prevention is not a realistic goal; most patients with Alzheimer's disease will suffer repeated episodes of delirium. Attention to the following guidelines for medical care of patients with Alzheimer's disease can minimize the incidence and morbidity of delirium.

- Nonpharmacological therapy is often safer and more effective than drug therapy.

  This is particularly true for musculoskeletal problems. Many clinicians prescribe nonsteroidal anti-inflammatory drugs whenever their patients complain of aches and pains. However, the main use of these drugs should be for the treatment of true inflammation (e.g., gout). Mechanical neck and back pain, almost universally present in elderly patients, can be more effectively treated with heat and exercise. Foot pain responds better to appropriate orthotics than to medications.

- When drug therapy is necessary, medications that act locally or are minimally absorbed are preferable.

  Carafate or antacids are much safer than histamine H_2 receptor blockers. A steroid preparation injected directly into the site of an inflamed bursa is more effective and safer than oral nonsteroidal anti-inflammatory therapy. Inhaled bronchodilators are more effective and less toxic in the treatment of bronchospasm than systemically administered agents.

- When systemic drugs are used, start with low doses and titrate up slowly.

  For reasons outlined earlier, the appropriate dose of drugs for this population is often impossible to predict. Unless the need for treatment is urgent, caution is indicated. This is particularly important for psychotropic drugs, which commonly cause adverse cognitive and behavioral effects.

- Within a class of drugs, choose agents with minimal activity in the CNS.

  When histamine H_2 receptor blockers are necessary to treat active peptic ulcer disease, ranitidine is preferable to cimetidine. Among beta-adrenergic receptor blockers, atenolol is safer than propranolol.

- When prescribing psychotropic drugs, choose agents with the least anticholinergic activity.

  Among tricyclic antidepressants, nortriptyline and desipramine are much less likely to cause delirium than amitriptyline and imipramine. Haloperidol, the neuroleptic with the least anticholinergic effect, is usually preferable to lower-potency drugs such as thioridazine and chlorpromazine.

- Whenever medications are prescribed for patients with Alzheimer's disease, the clinician should be committed to serial quantitative assessments of the cognitive and behavioral effects of the drugs.

To monitor potential adverse consequences of drug therapy, repeated evaluations should be made, with tools such as the MMSE for cognitive function and attention and the Brief Psychiatric Rating Scale (Overall and Gorham 1962) for behavioral symptoms. Reliance on casual, qualitative assessment is likely to result in delayed recognition of toxicity.

- Even in the absence of demonstrable toxicity, drugs should be discontinued when the benefits are not evident.

  For example, a nonsteroidal anti-inflammatory drug prescribed for inflammatory pain should be continued only if it is providing definite benefit. Usually the only way to assess the benefit is to discontinue the drug to see whether symptoms worsen.

- When an Alzheimer's disease patient deteriorates, consider drug toxicity first. Minimize systemic drugs, and investigate possible medical comorbidities before prescribing additional psychotropic drugs.

There is no area in which cooperation between internist and psychiatrist is more critical than in the evaluation and management of behavioral complications in patients with dementia. In the preface to their book on delirium, Lindesay and colleagues (1990) noted that frequently, problems of the diagnosis and management of delirium become battles between physicians and psychiatrists over "difficult" patients. In these challenging cases, optimal outcomes require a multidisciplinary approach, with careful attention to clinical detail and thoughtful judgment regarding therapeutic interventions. Collaboration between internist and psychiatrist should occur before a diagnosis is established and also before a treatment plan is initiated.

References

Adler S: Methyldopa-induced decrease in mental activity. JAMA 230:1428–1429, 1974

American Psychiatric Association: Diagnostic and Statistical Manual of Mental Disorders, 4th Edition. Washington, DC, American Psychiatric Association, 1994

Anthony JC, LeResche L, Niaz V, et al: Limits of the "Mini-Mental State" as a screening test for dementia and delirium among hospital patients. Psychol Med 12:397–408, 1982

Bigger JT: Digitalis toxicity. J Clin Pharmacol 25:514–521, 1985

Blass JP, Nolan KA, Black RS, et al: Delirium: phenomenology and diagnosis—a neurobiologic view. Int Psychogeriatr 3:121–134, 1991

Brenner RP: Utility of EEG in delirium: past views and current practice. Int Psychogeriatr 3:211–229, 1991

Burrows J, Briggs RS, Elkington AR: Cataract extraction and confusion in elderly patients. Journal of Clinical and Experimental Gerontology 7:51–70, 1985

Davidson J: The pharmacologic treatment of psychiatric disorders in the elderly, in Geriatric Psychiatry. Edited by Busse EW, Blazer DG. Washington, DC, American Psychiatric Press, 1992, pp 515–542

Drachman DA, Leavitt J: Human memory and the cholinergic system. Arch Neurol 30:113–121, 1974

Drugs that may cause psychiatric symptoms. The Medical Letter 31:113–118, 1989

Engel GL, Romano J: Delirium, a syndrome of cerebral insufficiency. Journal of Chronic Diseases 4:260–276, 1959

Evans LK: "Sundown syndrome" in institutionalized elderly. J Am Geriatr Soc 35:101–108, 1987

Folstein M, Folstein S, McHugh P: Mini-Mental State: a practical method for grading the cognitive state of patients for the clinician. J Psychiatr Res 12:189–198, 1975

Hobson JA, Lydic R, Baghodoyan HA: Evolving concepts of sleep cycle generation: from brain centers to neuronal populations. Behavioral Brain Science 9:371–448, 1986

Houston MC: Clonidine hydrochloride: review of pharmacologic and clinical aspects. Progr Cardiovasc Dis 23:337–350, 1981

Husserl FE, Messerli FH: Adverse effects of antihypertensive drugs. Drugs 22:188–210, 1981

Jarvik MA: Antidepressant therapy for the geriatric patient. J Clin Psychopharmacol 1:55S–61S, 1981

Jenike MA: Geriatric Psychiatry and Psychopharmacology: A Clinical Approach. Chicago, IL, Year Book Medical, 1989, pp 215–230

Karhunen U, Raitta C: Psychiatric reactions complicating intracapsular cataract surgery: a prospective study. Ophthalmic Surg 13:1008–1112, 1982

Koponen H, Stenback U, Mattila E, et al: CSF beta-endorphin immunore-activity in delirium. Biol Psychiatry 25:938–944, 1989

Kral VA: Confused states: descriptiion and management, in Modern Perspectives in the Psychiatry of Old Age. Edited by Howells JG. New York, Brunner/Mazel, 1975, pp 356–362

Kramp P, Bolwig TG: Electroconvulsive therapy in acute delirious states. Compr Psychiatry 22:368–371, 1981

Lindesay J, MacDonald A, Starke I: Delirium in the Elderly. Oxford, England, Oxford University Press, 1990, pp 66–79

Lipowski ZJ: Delirium in the elderly patient. N Engl J Med 320:578–582, 1989

Lipowski ZJ: Delirium: Acute Confusional States, 2nd Edition. New York, Oxford University Press, 1990, pp 141–174

Manepalli J, Grossberg GT, Mueller C: Prevalence of delirium and urinary tract infection in a psychogeriatric unit. J Geriatr Psychiatry Neurol 3:198–202, 1990

Meyer BR: Benzodiazepines in the elderly. Med Clin North Am 66:1017–1035, 1982

Overall JE, Gorham DR: The Brief Psychiatric Rating Scale. Psychol Rep 10:799–812, 1962

Perry EK, Johnson M, Kerwin JM, et al: Convergent cholinergic activities in aging and Alzheimer's disease. Neurobiol Aging 13:393–400, 1992

Phelps ME, Mazziotta JC, Huang SC: Study of cerebral function with positron emission tomography. J Cereb Blood Flow Metab 2:113–162, 1982

Rabins PV, Folstein MF: Delirium and dementia: diagnostic and fatality rates. Br J Psychol 140:149–153, 1982

Roberts AH: The value of ECT in delirium. Br J Psychiatry 109:653–655, 1963

Salzman C, Shader RL, Greenblatt DJ, et al: Long versus short half-life benzodiazepines in the elderly. Arch Gen Psychiatry 40:293–297, 1983

Sorock GS, Shimkin EE: Use of benzodiazepine sedatives and risk of falling in a community-dwelling elderly cohort. Arch Intern Med 148:2441–2444, 1988

Tinetti ME, Speechley M, Guiter SF: Risk factors for falls among elderly persons living in the community. N Engl J Med 319:1701–1707, 1988

Tune LE, Bylsma FW: Benzodiazepine-induced and anticholinergic-induced delirium in the elderly. Int Psychogeriatr 3:397–408, 1991

CHAPTER 5

Possible Neurobiological Basis for Behavioral Symptoms

Brian A. Lawlor, M.D., F.R.C.P.I., M.R.C.Psych.

Alzheimer's disease is the most common cause of dementia, afflicting at least 3–4 million Americans. Marked behavioral and mood changes can accompany the inexorable cognitive deterioration in Alzheimer's disease, with the development of aggression, agitation, paranoia, hallucinations, sleep disturbance, and/or depression in more than 50% of both community-based and nursing home patients (Reisberg et al. 1987; Swearer et al. 1988). In contrast to the core cognitive symptoms, which usually follow a well-described course, the occurrence and course of these noncognitive symptoms in Alzheimer's disease are not so predictable (Teri et al. 1988) and may develop at any stage during the disease process (Eisdorfer et al. 1992).

It is these behavioral disturbances, rather than the memory loss, that make caring for these patients difficult and often impossible at times. Furthermore, behavioral complications are a leading cause of hospitalization and institutionalization in Alzheimer's disease patients (Steele et al. 1990), and their presence, particularly in the case of psychosis, may predict a more rapid rate of decline (Drevets and Rubin 1989; Mayeux et al. 1985).

Over the past 10 years, data have accumulated regarding the

possible neurotransmitter basis for the cognitive and behavioral changes associated with Alzheimer's disease. Much of this evidence points to the importance of cholinergic system abnormalities as the basis for memory and cognitive difficulties associated with the disease (Coyle et al. 1983; Davies and Maloney 1976; Whitehouse et al. 1982). The so-called cholinergic hypothesis has led to many pharmacological attempts to enhance cholinergic transmission in Alzheimer's disease (Davis and Mohs 1986; Summers et al. 1986). The cholinergic abnormalities in Alzheimer's disease, however, do not occur in isolation; defects in other neurotransmitter systems, such as the noradrenergic, serotonergic, and dopaminergic systems also occur and may contribute to the core cognitive symptoms of Alzheimer's disease.

The added presence of monoaminergic deficits in this disease may therefore explain the failure of cholinomimetic therapy to significantly improve cognition in most patients. Monoaminergic dysfunction in Alzheimer's disease may also contribute to the expression of the behavioral problems in these patients. In this chapter, the evidence supporting a relationship between behavioral symptoms and monoaminergic system dysfunction in Alzheimer's disease is discussed.

Evidence for Monoaminergic Abnormalities in Alzheimer's Disease

Norepinephrine

There is both neuropathological and biochemical evidence of significant abnormalities in the noradrenergic system in Alzheimer's disease (Bondareff et al. 1982; Perry et al. 1981). Postmortem studies have demonstrated decreased numbers of neurons in the locus coeruleus of patients with Alzheimer's disease (Bondareff et al. 1982; Chan-Palay and Asan 1989; Forstyl et al. 1992; Mann et al. 1984; Zweig et al. 1988). Brain norepinephrine (NE) levels in Alzheimer's disease patients have also been found to be decreased compared with those in control subjects (Adolfsson et al. 1979; Baker and Reynolds 1989; Zubenko et al. 1990) and the levels of the NE metabolite 3-methoxy-4-hydroxyphenylglycol (MHPG) to be increased (Gottfries et al. 1983). Studies of cerebrospinal fluid (CSF) and plasma have demonstrated both NE and MHPG levels to be increased in Alzheimer's disease patients (Raskind et al. 1984; Winblad et al. 1982), possibly reflecting increased turnover of NE in the periphery. Peripheral changes could of course be secondary to behavioral problems, such as agitation, so frequently observed in these patients.

Further evidence for a significant noradrenergic deficit in Alzheimer's disease is the fact that the levels of dopamine-beta-hydroxylase, the enzyme involved in the synthesis of NE from dopamine and a marker of central noradrenergic function, have been found to be decreased in the frontal and temporal lobes and in the CSF of Alzheimer's disease patients compared with those in control subjects (Cross et al. 1981; Soininen et al. 1990).

Serotonin

A number of lines of evidence point to significant changes in the activity of the serotonergic system in Alzheimer's disease. Autopsy studies of the brains of patients with the disease have found decreased levels of 5-hydroxytryptamine (serotonin; 5-HT), and to a lesser extent 5-hydroxyindoleacetic acid (5-HIAA), in different cortical areas (Bowen et al. 1983; Cross et al. 1984, 1986). Other studies have found decreased levels of 5-HIAA in the CSF of patients with Alzheimer's disease, with the lowest levels in the more severely affected patients (Soininen et al. 1981). Receptor binding studies have also found marked reductions in cortical $5-HT_2$ receptors and to a lesser extent $5-HT_1$ receptors (Bowen et al. 1983; Cross et al. 1984, 1986). Presynaptic deficits, notably decreased 5-HT reuptake and release, have been demonstrated in biopsy specimens from patients with confirmed Alzheimer's disease (Palmer et al. 1987).

From a neuropathological point of view, greater cell loss and increased numbers of neurofibrillary tangles have also been found in the dorsal raphe nuclei of Alzheimer's disease patients compared with control subjects (Ishii 1986; Mann et al. 1984).

Dopamine

The clinical finding of extrapyramidal symptoms in up to 30% of Alzheimer's disease patients and the overlap of Parkinson's disease and Alzheimer's disease (Mayeux et al. 1985; Pearce 1974) are indirect indications of dopaminergic dysfunction, at least in a subgroup of Alzheimer's disease patients. Also indicative of significant damage to this neurotransmitter system in Alzheimer's disease are the presence of cytopathological changes in the substantia nigra (Ditter and Mirra 1987; Leverenz and Sumi 1986; Zubenko et al. 1990), decreases in brain dopamine and homovanillic acid (HVA) (Adolfsson et al. 1979; Gottfries et al. 1983; Gottfries et al. 1986), and reductions in CSF HVA levels (Brane et al. 1989; Gottfries et al. 1974; Parnetti et al. 1987; Soininen et al. 1981).

Possible Neurotransmitter Basis for Behavioral Change in Alzheimer's Disease

Norepinephrine

A number of recent studies have found decreased postmortem locus coeruleus cell counts in Alzheimer's disease patients who had a history of depression (Chan-Palay and Asan 1989; Forstyl et al. 1992; Zubenko et al. 1988; Zweig et al. 1988). Furthermore, cortical NE levels are also significantly decreased in depressed Alzheimer's disease patients compared with those in nondepressed Alzheimer's disease patients (Zubenko and Moossy 1990).

In contrast to depression, in postmortem examination of Alzheimer's disease patients with psychosis, raised or relatively preserved NE levels have been found in the substantia nigra and other brain areas (Zubenko et al. 1991). A weak association was also found between central measures of noradrenergic function and increased agitation: CSF MHPG correlated with measures of restlessness in Alzheimer's disease patients (Brane et al. 1989). Furthermore, an association between CSF MHPG and increased severity of dementia (Raskind et al. 1984) could reflect increased agitation in these more severely affected patients.

Serotonin

Depression in Alzheimer's disease has been associated with a significant loss of 5-HT neurons in the raphe nuclei (Zubenko et al. 1988; Zweig et al. 1988), and there is a tendency for 5-HT to be decreased in most brain areas in depressed Alzheimer's disease patients (Zubenko et al. 1990). With regard to the occurrence of psychotic symptoms in Alzheimer's disease, there is a reported decrease in 5-HT in the prosubiculum in patients with a history of psychotic symptoms compared with nonpsychotic patients (Zubenko et al. 1991).

These findings suggest that the development of depression and psychosis in Alzheimer's disease may be associated with a serotonergic deficit. However, the data supporting a relationship between 5-HT and depression in Alzheimer's disease are relatively weaker than those noted for norepinephrine and depression (Zubenko et al. 1990), and further studies in this area are indicated.

With regard to agitation, a single postmortem study found a relationship between decreases in cortical 5-HT and agitated behavior (Palmer et al. 1988), suggesting a possible serotonergic basis for this behavioral disturbance in Alzheimer's disease.

Anxiety has also been linked to changes in 5-HT function in patients with Alzheimer's disease; one study found a positive correlation between anxiety and 5-HIAA levels (Brane et al. 1989).

Pharmacological probe studies with the selective serotonin agonist *m*-chlorophenylpiperazine (*m*-CPP) in Alzheimer's disease also provide indirect evidence for a relationship between behavioral disturbances and altered serotonin function. Alzheimer's disease patients show greater behavioral responses when challenged with *m*-CPP compared with age-matched control subjects, suggesting that a hyperresponsive 5-HT system in Alzheimer's disease could account for the frequent occurrence of behavioral disturbances in this illness (Lawlor et al. 1989).

Dopamine

Changes in the dopaminergic system in Alzheimer's disease have been implicated in the etiology of some of the behavioral disturbances, as well as in the development of motoric changes that accompany this illness. With regard to depression, greater cytopathology in the substantia nigra was found in patients with major depression, although there were no significant changes in the dopamine levels of the substantia nigra compared with those of nondepressed Alzheimer's disease patients (Zubenko et al. 1990). Decreased CSF HVA levels were associated with greater depression in some studies (Gottfries et al. 1983) but not in others (Brane et al. 1989). Interestingly, no association has been found between psychotic symptoms and changes in central dopamine function in Alzheimer's disease. Clearly, further study of the role of the dopaminergic pathway in depression and in other behavioral symptoms in Alzheimer's disease is warranted.

Because of the association between the parkinsonian type of symptoms in Alzheimer's disease patients (Mayeux et al. 1985; Pearce 1974) and the fact that Parkinson's disease is caused by central dopaminergic dysfunction, it is attractive to theorize a role for dopamine in the development of similar symptoms in Alzheimer's disease patients (Gottfries et al. 1983). In support of this hypothesis, a significant negative association was demonstrated between CSF HVA levels and impaired motor function in Alzheimer's disease (Brane et al. 1989; Kaye 1988).

Implications for Treatment

So far, drug treatments for behavioral disturbances have been empirically based, are ineffective in a significant proportion of patients, and produce problematic side effects. An understanding of the neurobiological basis for some of these disturbing symptoms may aid the development of new and improved agents in this area.

Preliminary evidence already exists that targeted therapies addressing the neurotransmitter imbalance in Alzheimer's disease might be helpful. For example, selegiline, a monoamine oxidase type B (MAO-B) selective inhibitor, has been tried in Alzheimer's disease because there is evidence of increased brain MAO-B activity in this disease (Adolffson et al. 1979). A number of studies have demonstrated improvement in behavior with this agent, specifically increased socialization and interaction and decreased energy and depressive symptoms (Lawlor et al. 1992; Tariot et al. 1987). This finding of improvement is in keeping with the demonstrated relationship between amotivation, depression, and decreased measures of dopamine function in Alzheimer's disease (Brane et al. 1989; Gottfries 1980).

Other preliminary evidence in support of this hypothesis is the efficacy of the selective serotonin reuptake inhibitor citalopram in decreasing emotionality and improving behavior in Alzheimer's disease patients (Nyth and Gottfries 1990), suggesting that the enhancement of 5-HT function in Alzheimer's disease can have ameliorative effects on behavior in this condition. In this situation, citalopram may be acting to down-regulate a hypersensitive 5-HT system that, as suggested earlier (Lawlor et al. 1989), may be contributing to the clinical expression of behavioral disturbance in Alzheimer's disease.

An understanding of the neurotransmitter dysfunction associated with Alzheimer's disease can also be helpful in predicting the side effect profile of potential pharmacotherapeutic agents used to treat behavioral symptoms in this disorder. Alzheimer's disease patients are twice as sensitive to the cognitive impairment effects of the muscarinic antagonist scopolamine as are control subjects (Sunderland et al. 1987). This sensitivity, a result of the profound cholinergic lesion in Alzheimer's disease, indicates that psychotropic agents with potent anticholinergic properties will be poorly tolerated by this patient population. Alzheimer's disease patients also develop extrapyramidal side effects at low doses of neuroleptics. These patients can rarely tolerate doses greater than 2–3 mg of haloperidol per day without developing pseudoparkinsonism (Devanand et al. 1989), a symptom most likely due to the presence of dopaminergic deficits in some Alzheimer's disease patients. Because of this increased sensitivity to dopamine and cholinergic blockade, the ideal antipsychotic for Alzheimer's disease patients must have low potential for extrapyramidal side effects and minimal anticholinergic properties. Fortunately, the development of new agents with a 5-HT$_2$/D$_2$ profile may result in fewer extrapyramidal side effects and should be helpful for Alzheimer's disease patients with psychotic symptoms.

Conclusions

There is evidence from clinicopathological studies that depression in Alzheimer's disease may be associated with changes in the noradrenergic and, to a lesser extent, the dopaminergic and serotonergic systems. These findings represent the first demonstration of a relationship between pathological or neurochemical changes in monoaminergic systems and the presence of neuropsychiatric symptoms. Weak links have also been found between agitation and postmortem changes in serotonergic function, although further work in this area is indicated. Preliminary studies using pharmacological probes in living Alzheimer's disease patients implicate 5-HT dysfunction in a broad range of behavioral disturbances, which may be ameliorated with selective 5-HT agents. Future developments will expand our knowledge of the possible neurotransmitter basis for some of the behavioral symptoms in Alzheimer's disease and may lead to more effective and better tolerated pharmacological therapies for specific behavioral disturbances in this disease.

References

Adolfsson R, Gottfries CG, Roos BE, et al: Changes in the brain catecholamines in patients with dementia of the Alzheimer type. Br J Psychiatry 135:2196–2223, 1979

Baker GB, Reynolds GP: Biogenic amines and their metabolites in Alzheimer's disease: noradrenaline, 5-hydroxytryptamine and 5-hydroxyindole-3-acetic acid depleted in hippocampus but not in substantia innominata. Neurosci Lett 100:335–339, 1989

Bondareff W, Mountjoy CQ, Roth M: Loss of neurons of origin of the adrenergic projection to the cerebral cortex (nucleus locus coeruleus) in senile dementia. Neurology 32:164–168, 1982

Bowen DM, Allen SJ, Benton JS, et al: Biochemical assessment of serotonergic and cholinergic dysfunction and cerebral atrophy and Alzheimer's disease. J Neurochem 41:266–272, 1983

Brane G, Gottfries CG, Blennow K, et al: Monoamine metabolites in cerebrospinal fluid and behavioral ratings in patients with early and late onset of Alzheimer's disease. Alzheimer Dis Assoc Disord 3:148–156, 1989

Chan-Palay V, Asan E: Alterations in catecholamine neurons of the locus coeruleus in senile dementia of the Alzheimer type and in Parkinson's disease with and without dementia and depression. J Comp Neurol 287:373–392, 1989

Coyle JT, Price DL, DeLong MR: Alzheimer's disease: a disorder of cortical cholinergic innervation. Science 219:1184–1190, 1983

Cross AJ, Crow TJ, Perry EK, et al: Reduced dopamine-beta-hydroxylase activity in Alzheimer's disease. BMJ 1:93–94, 1981

Cross AJ, Crow TJ, Ferrier IN, et al: Serotonin receptor changes in dementia of the Alzheimer type. J Neurochem 53:1574–1581, 1984

Cross AJ, Crow TJ, Ferrier IN, et al: The selectivity of the reduction of S2 receptors in Alzheimer type dementia. Neurobiol Aging 7:3–7, 1986

Davies P, Maloney AFJ: Selective loss of central cholinergic neurons in Alzheimer's disease. Lancet 2:1403, 1976

Davis KL, Mohs RC: Cholinergic drugs in Alzheimer's disease. N Engl J Med 315:1286–1287, 1986

Devanand DP, Sackeim HA, Brown R, et al: A pilot study of haloperidol treatment of psychosis and behavioral disturbance in Alzheimer's disease. Arch Neurol 46:854–857, 1989

Ditter SM, Mirra SS: Neuropathologic and clinical features of Parkinson's disease in Alzheimer's disease patients. Neurology 37:754–760, 1987

Drevets WC, Rubin EH: Psychotic symptoms and the longitudinal course of senile dementia of the Alzheimer type. Biol Psychiatry 25:39–48, 1989

Eisdorfer C, Cohen D, Paveza GJ, et al: An empirical evaluation of the Global Deterioration Scale for staging Alzheimer's disease. Am J Psychiatry 149:190–194, 1992

Forstyl H, Burns A, Luthert P, et al: Clinical and neuropathological correlates of depression in Alzheimer's disease. Psychol Med 22:877–884, 1992

Gottfries CG: Biochemistry of dementia and normal ageing. Trends Neurosci 3:55–57, 1980

Gottfries CG, Kjallqvist A, Ponten U, et al: Cerebrospinal fluid pH and monoamine and glycolytic metabolites in Alzheimer's disease. Br J Psychiatry 124:280–287, 1974

Gottfries CG, Adolfsson R, Aquilonius SM, et al: Biochemical changes in dementia disorders of Alzheimer type (AD/SDAT). Neurobiol Aging 4:261–271, 1983

Gottfries CG, Bartfai T, Carlsson A, et al: Multiple biochemical deficits in both gray and white matter of Alzheimer brains. Prog Neuropsychopharmacol Biol Psychiatry 10:405–413, 1986

Ishii T: Distribution of Alzheimer's neurofibrillary changes in the brain stem and hypothalamus of senile dementia. Acta Neuropathol 6:181–187, 1986

Kaye J: Neurochemical aspects of motor impairment, in Alzheimer Disease: Clinical and Biological Heterogeneity (panel). Moderated by Friedland RP. Ann Intern Med 109:307–308, 1988

Lawlor BA, Sunderland T, Mellow AM, et al: Hyperresponsivity to the serotonin agonist meta-chlorophenylpiperazine (m-CPP) in Alzheimer's disease: a controlled study. Arch Gen Psychiatry 46:542–549, 1989

Lawlor BA, Greene C, Aisen PS: Selegiline improves behavioral symptoms in Alzheimer's disease. Paper presented at the Collegium Internationale Neuro-Psychopharmacologium (CINP) XVIIIth Congress, Nice, Italy, June 28–July 2, 1992

Leverenz J, Sumi MS: Parkinson's disease in patients with Alzheimer's disease. Arch Neurol 43:662–664, 1986

Mann DMA, Yates PI, Marcyniuk B: A comparison of changes in the nucleus basalis and the locus coeruleus in Alzheimer's disease. J Neurol Neurosurg Psychiatry 47:201–203, 1984

Mayeux R, Stern Y, Spanton S: Heterogeneity in dementia of the Alzheimer type: evidence for subgroups. Neurology 35:453–461, 1985

Nyth AL, Gottfries CG: The clinical efficacy of citalopram in treatment of emotional disturbance in dementia disorders: a Nordic multicentre study. Br J Psychiatry 157:894–901, 1990

Palmer AM, Francis PT, Benton JS, et al: Presynaptic serotonergic dysfunction in patients with Alzheimer's disease. J Neurochem 48:8–15, 1987

Palmer AM, Statman GC, Procter AW, et al: Possible neurotransmitter basis of behavioral changes in Alzheimer's disease. Ann Neurol 34:616–620, 1988

Parnetti L, Gottfries J, Karlsson I, et al: Monoamine metabolites in cerebrospinal fluid of patients with senile dementia of the Alzheimer type using high performance liquid chromatography and gas chromatography–mass spectrometry. Acta Psychiatr Scand 75:542–548, 1987

Pearce J: Mental changes in parkinsonism (letter). BMJ 1:445, 1974

Perry EK, Tomlinson BE, Blessed G, et al: Neuropathological and biochemical observations on the noradrenergic system in Alzheimer's disease. J Neurol Sci 51:279–287, 1981

Raskind MA, Peskind ER, Halter JB, et al: Norepinephrine and MHPG levels in CSF and plasma in Alzheimer's disease. Arch Gen Psychiatry 41:343–346, 1984

Reisberg B, Borenstein J, Salob SP, et al: Behavioral symptoms in Alzheimer's disease: phenomenology and treatment. J Clin Psychiatry 48 (suppl):9–15, 1987

Soininen H, MacDonald E, Rekonen M, et al: Homovanillic acid and 5-hydroxyindoleacetic acid levels in cerebrospinal fluid of patients with senile dementia of Alzheimer type. Acta Neurol Scand 64:101–107, 1981

Soininen H, Pitkanen A, Halonen T, et al: Dopamine-beta-hydroxylase and acetylcholinesterase activity of cerebrospinal fluid in Alzheimer's disease. Acta Neurol Scand 69:29–34, 1990

Steele C, Rovner B, Chasse A, et al: Psychiatric symptoms and nursing home placement with Alzheimer's disease. Am J Psychiatry 147:1049–1051, 1990

Summers WK, Majovski LV, Marsh GM, et al: Oral tetrahydroaminoacridine in long-term treatment of senile dementia Alzheimer type. N Engl J Med 315:1241–1245, 1986

Sunderland T, Tariot PN, Cohen RM, et al: Anticholinergic sensitivity in patients with dementia of the Alzheimer type: a dose response study. Arch Gen Psychiatry 44:418–426, 1987

Swearer JM, Drachman DA, O' Donnell BF, et al: Troublesome and disruptive behaviors in dementia. J Am Geriatr Soc 36:784–790, 1988

Tariot PN, Cohen RM, Sunderland T, et al: L-Deprenyl in Alzheimer's disease. Arch Gen Psychiatry 44:427–433, 1987

Teri L, Larson EB, Reifler BV: Behavioral disturbance in dementia of the Alzheimer's type. J Am Geriatr Soc 36:1–6, 1988

Winblad B, Adolfsson R, Carlsson A, et al: Biogenic amines in brains of patients with Alzheimer's disease, in Alzheimer's Disease: A Report of Progress in Research. Edited by Corkin S, Davis KL, Growdon JH, et al. New York, Raven, 1982, pp 25–33

Whitehouse PJ, Price DL, Struble RG, et al: Alzheimer's disease and senile dementia—loss of neurons in the basal forebrain. Science 215:1237–1239, 1982

Zubenko GS, Moossy J: Major depression in primary dementia: clinical and neuropathological correlates. Arch Neurol 45:1182–1186, 1988

Zubenko GS, Moossy J, Kopp U: Neurochemical correlates of major depression in primary dementia. Arch Neurol 47:209–214, 1990

Zubenko GS, Moossy J, Martinez AJ, et al: Neuropathological and neurochemical correlates of psychosis in primary dementia. Arch Neurol 48:619–623, 1991

Zweig RM, Ross CA, Hedreen JC, et al: The neuropathology of aminergic nuclei in Alzheimer's disease. Ann Neurol 24:233–242, 1988

CHAPTER 6

Measurement of Behavioral Changes

John T. Little, M.D.
Susan E. Molchan, M.D.
Marc Cantillon, M.D.
Trey Sunderland, M.D.

Whereas cognitive functioning is usually the central focus of Alzheimer's disease research, it is behavioral symptoms that frequently determine the level of care required for the clinical management of individual patients. Furthermore, as more information has become available about the multineurotransmitter nature of Alzheimer's disease pathology, the interaction of behavioral and cognitive abnormalities takes on more importance from a research perspective as well. In light of the increased prominence of behavioral symptoms, rating scales designed to measure change in such symptoms have become central to clinical research in Alzheimer's disease. In this chapter we review and critique the growing field of behavioral assessment in Alzheimer's disease. For this purpose, we have chosen 26 instruments published over the last 19 years that assess and quantify behavioral issues regarding Alzheimer's disease patients.

As noted in previous chapters, the manifestation of behavioral symptoms varies greatly among individuals with Alzheimer's disease. Furthermore, cognitive status and functional abilities are important influences on behavioral and psychiatric symptoms. Hence, the study of Alzheimer's disease patients will ideally use multiple instruments or measurements that are broad in scope, that include functional and cognitive data in addition to psychiatric symptoms, and that are valid and reliable over time. For the purpose of this review, *validity* refers to whether the scale actually measures what it is intended to measure; *reliability* refers to the scale's dependability with time or between raters. When attempts to assess the validity and reliability of a scale have been made, we note them.

Global Dementia Rating Scales

Some global dementia rating scales incorporate behavioral symptoms, functional status, and cognitive status into one scale. For example, in 1982, two global dementia rating scales were published that incorporate broad measures and provide staging of the illness. These scales are the Clinical Dementia Rating (CDR) and the Global Deterioration Scale (GDS).

Clinical Dementia Rating

The Clinical Dementia Rating (CDR) (Hughes et al. 1982), revised in 1984 and 1988, provides a global cognitive and functional evaluation of Alzheimer's disease patients and has good validity and reliability (Berg 1984, 1988). This scale provides a 5-point range (0, 0.5, 1, 2, 3) for the clinician to rate the patient, on the basis of an interview of the patient and the caregiver, in six domains: memory, orientation, judgment and problem solving, community affairs, home and hobbies, and personal care.

Global Deterioration Scale

The Global Deterioration Scale (GDS) (Reisberg et al. 1982) categorizes individuals with primary degenerative dementia into seven stages of cognitive, functional, and behavioral decline. Stage 1 represents no cognitive decline, stage 7 very severe cognitive decline. Initial studies demonstrated high validity and reliability for the GDS, and it became a widely used scale (Reisberg et al. 1988). However, a recent large multicenter study has identified several limitations of the GDS for Alzheimer's disease. First, psychiatric symptoms and functional impairment were found in all stages of the illness, but the GDS emphasizes their presence in the later stages. Second, the rate of change of dysfunction was found to be different from that originally described (Eisdorfer et al. 1992).

Measurement and Relationship of Separate Domains

The authors of the multicenter study point out that because a great deal of evidence supports the heterogeneity of Alzheimer's disease, the best approach may be to use separate scales to measure cognitive function, psychiatric symptoms, and functional status until improved multidimensional instruments are available. They recommend, for example, the use of the Mini-Mental State Exam (MMSE) for cognitive measurements, the Direct Assessment of Functional Status (DAFS) for functional assessment, and the Alzheimer's Disease Assessment Scale (ADAS) for behavioral dysfunction.

The relationship among behavioral symptoms, cognitive status, and functional status in Alzheimer's disease is complex and controversial. Because Alzheimer's disease involves all three domains—behavior, cognition, and functional status—some assessment in each area is important, even if behavioral disturbance is the primary research interest. It was shown, for example, that behavioral symptoms are most common when cognitive dysfunction is moderate to severe, but not very severe (Reisberg et al. 1989). Other investigators, studying a community population of Alzheimer's disease patients with moderately severe dementia, showed that behavioral problems were pervasive, but not related to cognitive or functional ability (Teri et al. 1989). Within this sample of community-dwelling patients with moderate dementia, 20%–43% manifested emotional or activity disturbance. Interestingly, age was more predictive of functional difficulty than was cognitive dysfunction. In another study (Teri et al. 1988), Alzheimer's disease patients with mild, moderate, and severe dementia were examined. Results indicated that the number of behavioral problems increased with cognitive impairment and that the types of problems varied with severity of dementia. In the discussion to follow, therefore, instruments for measurement of cognitive function and functional status are briefly discussed, then separate scales for behavioral and for psychiatric symptoms are examined in more detail.

Cognitive Measurement

Probably the most commonly used and widely studied cognitive assessment tool in geropsychiatry is the MMSE (Folstein et al. 1975). Although it tests cognitive function only, its research utility is considerable because it is quickly administered, has been widely used, and has shown high validity and reliability (Cockrell and Folstein 1988; Folstein et al. 1975; Giordani et al. 1990). Limitations of the MMSE may include a reduced sensitivity for right-hemisphere dysfunction and very mild cognitive dysfunction in general. In addition, the MMSE may overestimate deficits in individuals older than 60 years or those with less than 9 years of education (Naugle and Kawczak 1989). Other instruments to assess cognition are reviewed at length elsewhere (e.g., Baddeley et al. 1990; Christensen et al. 1990; Saxton and Swihart 1989; Schultz and Pato 1988; Spinnler and DellaSala 1988).

Functional Assessment

Because cognitive status and functional status are related but distinct aspects of Alzheimer's disease (Reed et al. 1989; Skurla et al. 1988), measurement of functional status is also important, but it is often overlooked in describing the overall clinical status of the patient. One of the problems in this area has been the relative paucity of functional rating instruments designed specifically for Alzheimer's disease subjects. Two such instruments are discussed here.

Direct Assessment of Functional Status (DAFS)

One functional scale for these patients is the Direct Assessment of Functional Status (DAFS) scale (Loewenstein et al. 1989). It provides measurements for the following functions: time orientation, communication, transportation, financial matters, shopping, grooming, and eating. Interrater and test-retest reliability measures were high, and validity was demonstrated with established measures of functional status.

Daily Activities Questionnaire (DAQ)

The Daily Activities Questionnaire (DAQ) (Oakley et al. 1991) is another comprehensive functional assessment device designed specifically for use with these patients. This scale involves input from family, nursing staff, and an occupational therapist. Twelve areas of functioning are assessed, including personal and instrumental activities of daily living such as bathing, phone use, shopping, and cooking. Further discussion of functional assessment in Alzheimer's disease would be valuable, but it is beyond the scope of this chapter. (For reviews, see Fisher 1994; Kane and Kane 1981.)

General Behavioral Scales

Sandoz Clinical Assessment—Geriatric (SCAG)

The Sandoz Clinical Assessment—Geriatric (SCAG) (Shader et al. 1974, 1988) is one of the earliest clinician-rated instruments designed to evaluate global psychiatric symptoms in elderly people, and it has been shown to be reliable and valid (Overall and Rhoades 1988).

Behavioral Pathology in Alzheimer's Disease Rating Scale (BEHAVE-AD)

The Behavioral Pathology in Alzheimer's Disease rating scale (BEHAVE-AD) is a global behavioral scale designed specifically for Alzheimer's disease patients (Reisberg et al. 1987a, 1987b). It consists of 25 items in seven categories and also includes a global rating item. The categories include paranoia and delusions (items 1–7), hallucinations (8–12), activity disturbance (13–15), aggression (16–18), sleep disturbance (19), mood (20–21), and anxiety (22–25). The purpose of the BEHAVE-AD is to measure behaviors that are clinically relevant to the caregivers of Alzheimer's disease patients and that are potentially remediable by medications.

Other general behavioral scales are examined in the discussion that follows and are summarized in Table 6–1.

Measurement of Depression

Although a number of subjective rating scales are available to assess affective states in individuals without dementia, these scales are not necessarily appropriate for dementia patients, because self-report capacity may be impaired. A number of newer instruments incorporate data from family or caregivers, in addition to data from a clinical interview or an extended observation period such as a hospitalization. Several scales described were developed specifically to measure depression in individuals with dementia, but more general behavioral scales such as the ADAS and the new Behavioral Rating Scale for Dementia (BRSD) from CERAD (the Consortium to Establish a Registry for Alzheimer's Disease) (Tariot et al., in press) also contain sections on affective signs and symptoms.

All the scales measuring depression are discussed in the following sections and summarized in Table 6–2.

Cornell Scale for Depression in Dementia

One scale designed specifically to measure affective states in dementia is the Cornell Scale for Depression in Dementia (Alexopoulos et al. 1988a). This scale provides a rating based on a brief interview with the patient and information from the patient's caregiver. In this scale, 19 items are scored on a 4-point scale. Categories include mood-related signs, behavioral disturbance, physical signs, cyclic functions, and ideational disturbance. The scale has been shown to be valid and reliable for subjects with dementia who are in the hospital or in nursing home settings, but it has not been validated for those residing in the community (Alexopoulos et al. 1988a). Of interest also is that this scale has been validated for use as well in elderly subjects without dementia (Alexopoulos et al. 1988b).

Table 6–1. General behavioral rating scales

Scale	Reference	Rater	Target subjects	Strengths	Weaknesses
Alzheimer's Disease Assessment Scale (ADAS)	Rosen et al. 1984	Clinician	AD patients	Includes behavioral and cognitive assessment	Behavioral assessment
Behavioral Pathology in Alzheimer's Disease Rating Scale (BEHAVE-AD)	Reisberg et al. 1987a, 1987b	Clinician	AD patients	Specific for common behavioral problems in AD	—[a]
Behavioral and Emotional Activities Manifested in Dementia Scale (BEAM-D)	Sinha et al. 1992	Clinician	Dementia patients	Assessment of agitation	Less useful for mild dementia
CERAD Behavior Rating Scale for Dementia (BRSD)	Tariot et al. (in press)	Clinician	Dementia patients	Provides comprehensive assessment of psychopathology	Rating based only on caregivers' reports
Multidimensional Observation Scale for Elderly Subjects (MOSES)	Helmes et al. 1987	Nursing staff	Institution-alized elderly	Requires only brief weekly rating	Has not been studied for specific use with AD
Neurobehavioral Rating Scale (NRS)	Levin et al. 1987, Sultzer et al. 1992	Clinician	Head injury and dementia	Similar to BPRS	Interrater reliability not established for dementia

(continued)

Table 6–1. General behavioral rating scales (*continued*)

Scale	Reference	Rater	Target subjects	Strengths	Weaknesses
Revised Memory and Behavior Problem Checklist (RMBPC)	Teri et al. 1992	Caregiver	Dementia patients	Quantifies caregiver's reaction, has depression and agitation subscales	Relies only on caregivers
Sandoz Clinical Assessment—Geriatric (SCAG)	Shader et al. 1974	Clinician	Elderly	Broadly assesses psychopathology, including cognition	Deficient for psychosis and agitation

Note: AD, Alzheimer's disease.
[a] Empty cell indicates no weaknesses found.

Table 6–2. Depression scales

Scale	Reference	Rater	Target subjects	Strengths	Weaknesses
Alzheimer's Disease Assessment Scale (ADAS)[a]	Rosen et al. 1984	Clinician	Alzheimer's disease patients	Useful for mild to severe dementia	Only part of scale specific for depression
CERAD Behavior Rating Scale for Dementia (BRSD)	Tariot et al. (in press)	Clinician	Dementia patients	Quantifies frequency of behaviors	Rating based only on caregiver's report
Cornell Scale for Depression in Dementia	Alexopoulos et al. 1988a	Clinician	Dementia patients	Specific for depression in dementia	Not validated for outpatients
Depressive Signs Scale (DSS)	Katona and Aldridge 1985	Clinician	Dementia patients	Useful for severe dementia	Less descriptive for mild dementia
NIMH Dementia Mood Assessment Scale (DMAS)	Sunderland et al. 1988	Clinician	Dementia patients	Specific for depression in dementia	Not validated for severe dementia

[a]General behavioral rating scale.

Dementia Mood Assessment Scale (DMAS)

Another scale measuring affective symptoms in cognitively impaired individuals is the Dementia Mood Assessment Scale (DMAS) (Sunderland et al. 1988). It consists of 24 items covering four factors: depression, social interaction, anxiety, and vegetative symptoms. This scale is based on a clinical interview with the patient plus direct observation over time by staff. The DMAS requires that the patient be in a hospital or nursing home; it has been found valid and reliable for patients with probable Alzheimer's disease of mild to moderate severity. Like the Cornell scale, the DMAS serves to quantify affective signs and symptoms rather than to provide a diagnosis.

Scales for Affective Symptoms in More Severe Dementia

For Alzheimer's disease patients with more severe dementia, the Alzheimer's Disease Assessment Scale and the Depressive Signs Scale are useful in assessing affective symptoms.

Alzheimer's Disease Assessment Scale (ADAS).   Although only a limited part of the Alzheimer's Disease Assessment Scale (ADAS) (Rosen et al. 1984) pertains to affective signs and symptoms (less than half of 21 items), it is useful because it relies on an interview with the patient and with the relative or caregiver rather than on a self-report. Observations over the past week are incorporated into the following categories: tearfulness, depressed mood, concentration, cooperativeness, delusions, hallucinations, pacing, motor activity, tremors, and appetite. The ADAS was designed specifically for use with Alzheimer's disease patients, and reliability and validity have been established, but it is not intended to be a diagnostic instrument.

Depressive Signs Scale (DSS).   In a population with severe dementia the Depressive Signs Scale (DSS) (Katona and Aldridge 1985) is also useful for the assessment of depression (it was devised specifically for that purpose in a dexamethasone suppression study). The DSS contains nine items: sad appearance, agitation by day, slowness of movement, slowness of speech, early waking, loss of appetite, diurnal variation in mood, and interest in surroundings. Items are rated after a clinical interview with the patient and an interview with the nursing staff or a relative, based on the past week of activities. Interrater reliability is high, and the scale was validated with a depressed control group.

CERAD Behavior Rating Scale for Dementia (BRSD). A new scale with promise for measuring affective symptoms in dementia is the CERAD Behavior Rating Scale for Dementia (BRSD), created by the multicenter CERAD Clinical Task Force (Tariot et al., in press). The BRSD is a recently developed rater-administered, informant-based instrument. It assesses general behavioral functioning in dementia and contains a number of items relevant to depression. Preliminary analysis of the pilot study of 300 subjects suggests that the scale has high reliability and construct validity (Tariot 1992). The BRSD contains 51 items, scored on frequency rather than severity. For example, item 5 refers to crying by the subject. This can be scored as 0 (has never occurred), 1 (one to two times in past month), 2 (three to six times in past month), 3 (more than six times in past month), 8 (occurred since illness began, but not in past month), or 9 (unable to rate). It is hoped that the BRSD will eventually be used in diagnostic, therapeutic, correlative, and prognostic studies.

Measurement of Agitation

Another domain of behavioral disturbance in Alzheimer's disease for which measurement is desirable is agitated and disruptive behaviors (se also Chapter 1). As discussed in the section on affective disturbances, agitated behaviors can be measured by general behavioral scales as well as by several specific instruments currently available (see Table 6–3). Scales specifically designed to measure agitation include the Disruptive Behavior Rating Scales (DBRS), the Cohen-Mansfield Agitation Inventory (CMAI), the Brief Agitation Rating Scale (BARS), and the Agitated Behavior Mapping Instrument (ABMI). General behavioral scales that include components for agitation are numerous; more recent

Table 6–3.   Agitation scales

Scale	Reference	Rater	Target subjects	Strengths	Weaknesses
Agitated Behavior Mapping Instrument (ABMI)	Cohen-Mansfield et al. 1989b	Clinician	Dementia patients	Establishes behavior frequencies by direct observation	Use limited to skilled nursing facility
Behavioral and Emotional Activities Manifested in Dementia Scale (BEAM-D)[a]	Sinha et al. 1992	Clinician	Dementia patients	Based on interview of subject and caregiver	Does not assess general psychomotor activity
Brief Agitation Rating Scale (BARS)	Finkel et al. 1993	Clinician	Institutionalized elderly persons	Abbreviated version of CMAI; interrater reliability good	Further validation needed
Cohen-Mansfield Agitation Instrument (CMAI)	Cohen-Mansfield et al., 1986, 1989a, 1989c	Clinician	Dementia patients	Establishes behavior frequencies by direct observation	Use limited to skilled nursing facility; interrater reliability
Disruptive Behavior Rating Scales (DBRS)	Mungas et al. 1989	Clinician	Dementia patients	Data derived from multiple sources over several weeks	Use limited to skilled nursing facility
Multidimensional Observation Scale for Elderly Subjects (MOSES)[a]	Helmes et al. 1987	Nursing staff	Institutionalized elderly	Requires only brief weekly rating	Has not been studied for specific use with Alzheimer's disease

Neurobehavioral Rating Scale (NRS)[a]	Levin et al. 1987, Sultzer et al. 1992	Clinician	Patients with head injury and dementia	Rating similar to Brief Psychiatric Rating Scale (BPRS) based on single interview	Interrater reliability not established for dementia

[a] General behavioral rating scale.

examples include the Multidimensional Observation Scale for Elderly Subjects (MOSES), the Behavioral and Emotional Activities Manifested in Dementia Scale (BEAM-D), and the Neurobehavioral Rating Scale (NRS). Each of these scales is discussed below.

Disruptive Behavior Rating Scales (DBRS)

The Disruptive Behavior Rating Scales (DBRS) (Mungas et al. 1989) were developed to measure disruptive behaviors in four categories: physical aggression, verbal aggression, agitation, and wandering. A combined total disruptiveness score is derived by averaging the four components. This scale was designed for patients with dementia (particularly Alzheimer's disease) residing in a skilled nursing facility. Ratings begin with a daily checklist, completed by the nurse's aide assigned to the patient. The rater reviews the daily checklists as well as the patient's chart and interviews the relevant nursing staff before making a weekly rating. In addition, a nurse's assessment summary rating completed every 2–4 weeks provides additional data to the rater. Reliability is favorable for all scales of the DBRS. Validity measurements, however, were favorable for three scales but not for the verbal aggression scale. Nevertheless, this new scale focuses on clinically relevant disruptive behaviors in Alzheimer's disease patients, and with further study of the verbal aggression section, it holds promise as a highly useful scale.

Cohen-Mansfield Agitation Inventory (CMAI)

Another scale developed specifically to measure agitation is the Cohen-Mansfield Agitation Inventory (CMAI) (Cohen-Mansfield 1986; Cohen-Mansfield et al. 1989a, 1989c). This scale is a nurses' rating questionnaire listing 29 agitated behaviors. Each behavior is rated on a 7-point frequency scale from "never" to "several times per hour." This scale has been used for cognitively impaired individuals in a nursing home setting and can be used for around-the-clock ratings. Although the initial studies cited above demonstrated high interrater reliability, a recent study in another nursing home found only marginally adequate values (Finkel et al. 1992). Interrater reliability ratings calculated for subtypes of behaviors were .66 for physical aggression, .26 for nonaggressive physical behaviors, and .61 for verbal agitation. The same study did support the validity of the CMAI for measuring agitation.

Brief Agitation Rating Scale (BARS)

The Brief Agitation Rating Scale (BARS) is a new 10-item version of the CMAI, with better interrater reliability (Finkel et al. 1993). The intraclass correlation between rater pairs for the BARS was .73, compared to .41 for the CMAI. The authors suggested that the interrater reliability of the BARS is better because it includes the most salient and frequently observed behaviors from the CMAI. The validity of the BARS was supported in the same study.

Agitated Behavior Mapping Instrument (ABMI)

A scale similar to the CMAI is the Agitated Behavior Mapping Instrument (ABMI) (Cohen-Mansfield et al. 1989b), which was developed to study sundowning (the increased prevalence of psychiatric and behavioral symptoms in the early evening) in a unit of patients with Alzheimer's disease. This scale lists 25 agitated behaviors, which trained raters (research assistants) rated by frequency over a 3-minute observation period during each hour for 24 hours. Interrater reliability ratings for each behavior averaged .93.

Behavioral and Emotional Activities Manifested in Dementia (BEAM-D) Scale

A recently developed scale to assess behavioral agitation as well as other emotional disturbances in cognitively impaired elderly people is the Behavioral and Emotional Activities Manifested in Dementia (BEAM-D) Scale (Sinha et al. 1992). This scale consists of nine directly observed behaviors relevant to elderly dementia patients: hostility/aggression, destruction of property, disruption of others' activities, uncooperativeness, noncompliance, attention-seeking behavior, sexually inappropriate behavior, wandering, and hoarding. Seven inferred behaviors are also included on the scale: depression, delusions, hallucinations, anxiety, appropriateness, appetite, and insomnia. Scores are obtained after the rater interviews the patient and caregiver. Interrater reliability was high (.90), and validation with the Brief Psychiatric Rating Scale (BPRS) (Overall and Gorham 1962; Overall and Beller 1984) and the Sandoz Clinical Assessment—Geriatric (Shader et al. 1974) was established. The stated purpose for the development of the BEAM-D was to obtain a reliable scale for evaluation of drug treatments for behavioral problems in dementia. The authors also pointed out that this is a preliminary scale and that further research into its usefulness is ongoing. One deficiency of the scale is that there is no assessment of increased psychomotor activity such as pacing. Nevertheless, it is already a useful scale in assessing Alzheimer's disease patients with behavioral problems generally and agitation specifically.

Neurobehavioral Rating Scale (NRS)

Numerous general behavioral rating scales contain selected items on agitation. One general behavioral rating scale is the Neurobehavioral Rating Scale (NRS) (Levin et al. 1987). The NRS, a modified form of the BPRS, has been developed and validated for use in patients with dementia (Sultzer et al. 1992). The NRS is a 27-item scale that can be divided into six factors: cognition, agitation/disinhibition, behavioral retardation, anxiety/depression, language disturbance, and psychosis. (A 28th item, fluent aphasia, was added in the 1992 study cited above.) The NRS contains most of the items of the BPRS and is similarly scored by a trained rater after a structured interview with the patient. Although interrater reliability of the NRS has been established in patients with head injury, it has not yet been assessed for patients with dementia (Sultzer et al. 1992). Because the NRS is an observer-rated scale, establishing interrater reliability for use with Alzheimer's disease patients is an important task ahead.

Multidimensional Observation
Scale for Elderly Subjects (MOSES)

Another general behavioral scale, which includes a component on irritable behavior, or agitation, is the Multidimensional Observation Scale for Elderly Subjects (MOSES) (Helmes 1988; Helmes et al. 1987). This scale is used for institutionalized elderly patients and is rated by observers on the basis of activity over the previous week. It is best filled out by the nursing staff or the nurse's aides, because these individuals have the most direct day-to-day contact with the patient. The five areas of functioning (40 items) covered by this scale include self-care functioning, disoriented behavior, depressed/anxious mood, irritable behavior, and withdrawn behavior. Good reliability and validity measurements have been reported for the MOSES in a large sample of institutionalized elderly patients (Helmes et al. 1987), but the scale has not been studied for specific use with Alzheimer's disease.

Activity Monitors

A novel and very direct method of measuring physical agitation is the use of small electronic monitors of activity worn at the waist (Satlin et al. 1991; Teicher et al. 1986). The activity monitors were used to study circadian rhythms in institutionalized Alzheimer's disease patients with severe dementia by recording 5-minute epochs for 48–72 hours. An activity monitor containing solid-state memory was placed at waist level in the pocket of a vest worn over the subject's clothing. The hyperactivity of Alzheimer's disease patients who were pacers, as recorded on the activity monitors, corresponded to the clinical impressions of persistent activity and sleep fragmentation. These activity levels could also could be distinguished from those of Alzheimer's disease patients who were nonpacers and from those of an elderly control group (Satlin et al. 1991).

Measurement of Psychosis

Another important consequence of Alzheimer's disease that has behavioral features is psychosis. Several instruments designed to assess psychosis are discussed here.

Clinical Rating Scale for Psychosis in Alzheimer's Disease (SPAD)

The Clinical Rating Scale for Psychosis in Alzheimer's Disease (SPAD) is a nine-item scale developed specifically for psychotic symptoms common in Alzheimer's disease (Reisberg and Ferris

1985). Delusions of abandonment and delusions that "people are stealing things," as well as misidentification delusions, are specific items on the scale. Omissions from the scale include the misidentification delusion that one's own reflection is someone else and delusions of reference, which are not uncommon in Alzheimer's disease (Deutsch et al. 1991). Another possible shortcoming is that the final item on the scale, "other behavioral symptoms which may respond to neuroleptics," although inviting the inclusive scoring of any miscellaneous psychotic symptom, may lead to scoring error if a neuroleptic is prescribed inappropriately or is ineffective. Although this is clearly a useful scale, interrater reliability and test-retest reliability have not yet been established, to our knowledge.

Columbia University Scale for Psychopathology in Alzheimer's Disease (CUSPAD)

The Columbia University Scale for Psychopathology in Alzheimer's Disease (CUSPAD) (Devanand et al. 1992) is a new screening instrument designed to assess psychotic symptoms, although it also includes items pertaining to other behavioral disturbances. The scale includes operational definitions of delusions, hallucinations, and illusions that are common in Alzheimer's disease, and it allows scoring of frequency ("some of time" versus "most of time") and of whether the patient accepts the truth if corrected. Interrater reliability was established between a trained psychiatrist and a lay interviewer for 20 patients. The strength of this new scale is that it comprehensively contains 17 items of operationally defined psychotic symptoms that may be seen in Alzheimer's disease.

Behavioral Pathology in Alzheimer's Disease Rating Scale (BEHAVE-AD)

The BEHAVE-AD, a general behavioral scale discussed earlier in the chapter, can also be used to assess psychosis, because it contains a large number of relevant items (Reisberg et al. 1987a, 1987b).

Measurement of Personality Change

Although personality changes are common in Alzheimer's disease, there is to our knowledge no specific scale designed for the measurement of this consequence. The Neuroticism, Extraversion, Openness (NEO) Personality Inventory (Costa and McCrae 1985, 1988) was used in one study to examine personality changes in individuals with memory disorders (Seigler et al. 1991). In this study, the inventory (181 items) was filled out twice by the caregiver of the Alzheimer's disease patient, the first time to describe the premorbid personality and the second time the current personality of the Alzheimer's disease patient. A shorter scale, developed for head injury patients (Brooks and McKinlay 1983), was also used to study personality change in Alzheimer's disease patients (Petry et al. 1988, 1989). The same method has been used with this scale: the caregiver or spouse is asked to rate the Alzheimer's disease patient twice, regarding current and premorbid personality.

Family Assessments

As Alzheimer's disease patients deteriorate, their ability to serve as historian also declines; clinicians therefore rely progressively more on the caregiver or spouse to describe the patient's functioning. It is therefore reasonable to focus on assessment scales that rely on caregiver reporting in this review. It has been shown that family members and nursing staff may differ in their reporting of behavioral disturbances in Alzheimer's disease. Lukovits and McDaniel (1992) found that nurses reported more concern with vegetative behaviors such as incontinence, feeding, and sleep disturbance than did family members. There also tended to be disagreement between nurses and family members on behaviors that were difficult to define, such as depression, interest, and agitation. Three scales for relatives include the Relative's Assessment of Global Symptomatology, the Geriatric Evaluation by Relative's Rating Instrument, and the Revised Memory and Behavior Problems Checklist.

Relative's Assessment of Global Symptomatology (RAGS)

The Relative's Assessment of Global Symptomatology (RAGS) (Raskin and Crook 1988) contains 21 items relating to psychiatric symptoms and behavior in the community and is completed by a close friend or relative of the patient. This scale was not designed specifically for Alzheimer's disease patients, but rather for elderly psychiatric patients in general, which may include those with dementia and other disorders. Although the validity of the RAGS has been shown to be favorable, reliability has not been examined, to our knowledge.

Geriatric Evaluation by Relative's Rating Instrument (GERRI)

Another scale for relatives is the Geriatric Evaluation by Relative's Rating Instrument (GERRI) (Schwartz 1983, 1988). This scale has 49 items in three categories: cognitive functioning, social functioning, and mood. Items are rated on a 5-point frequency scale from "almost all of the time" to "almost never." Validity and reliability were shown in the initial study as well as in a more recent study, and this scale has been translated into a number of European and Asian languages (Schwartz 1988).

Revised Memory and Behavior Problems Checklist (RMBPC)

The Revised Memory and Behavior Problems Checklist (RMBPC) is a 24-item caregiver measure of behavioral problems in dementia patients (Teri et al. in press). The three subscales include depression, disruptive behaviors, and memory. Overall scale reliability and validity were good in the initial report. The RMBPC focuses on observable and potentially modifiable behaviors and evaluates the caregiver's reaction to each behavior. The checklist takes only about 10 minutes to complete. Because the RMBPC was designed specifically for dementia patients and emphasizes clinically relevant and practical problems, it is a welcome addition to existing instruments for evaluating general behavioral status as well as agitation and depression.

Conclusion

This review highlights some of the available instruments for the measurement of behavioral change in Alzheimer's disease. Behavioral scales can be global in their assessment of a broad range of psychiatric symptoms or more specific to syndromes such as depression or agitation. In addition to behavioral symptoms, scales are available for the measurement of cognitive and functional status, both independently and globally with behavioral status. The field has progressed so rapidly over the last few years that many scales have been designed specifically for Alzheimer's disease patients. Nevertheless, more work needs to be done in developing Alzheimer's disease scales that are more useful for descriptive and therapeutic studies. The collaborative development of the CERAD Rating Scale for Dementia represents one advance in the field that should significantly aid research. Further validation and reliability studies will help to elucidate the strengths and limitations of available instruments. Because the behavioral symptoms of Alzheimer's disease often dictate the level of care required and may help define clinical subtypes, improving the tools of measurement can only benefit clinical and research efforts.

References

Alexopoulos GS, Abrams RC, Young RC, et al: Cornell Scale for Depression in Dementia. Biol Psychiatry 23:271–284, 1988a

Alexopoulos GS, Abrams RC, Young RC, et al: Use of the Cornell scale in nondemented patients. J Am Geriatr Soc 36:230–236, 1988b

Baddeley A, DellaSala S, Spinnler H: The two-component hypothesis of memory deficit in Alzheimer's disease. J Clin Exp Neuropsychol 12:372–380, 1990

Berg L: Clinical Dementia Rating (correspondence). Br J Psychiatry 145:339, 1984

Berg L: Mild senile dementia of the Alzheimer type: diagnostic criteria and natural history. Mt Sinai J Med 55:87–96, 1988

Brooks KN, McKinlay W: Personality and behavioral change after severe blunt head injury: a relative's view. J Neurol Neurosurg Psychiatry 46:336–344, 1983

Christensen KJ, Multhaup KS, Ordstrom S, et al: Cognitive test profile analysis for the identification of dementia of the Alzheimer type. Alzheimer Dis Assoc Disord 4:96–109, 1990

Cockrell JR, Folstein MF: Mini-Mental State Examination (MMSE). Psychopharmacol Bull 24:689–692, 1988

Cohen-Mansfield J: Agitated behaviors in the elderly, II: preliminary results in the cognitively deteriorated. J Am Geriatr Soc 34:722–727, 1986

Cohen-Mansfield J, Marx MS, Rosenthal AS: A description of agitation in a nursing home. J Gerontol 44:M77–M84, 1989a

Cohen-Mansfield J, Watson V, Meade W, et al: Does sundowning occur in residents of an Alzheimer's unit? International Journal of Geriatric Psychiatry 4:293–298, 1989b

Cohen-Mansfield J, Werner P, Marx MS: An observational study of agitation in agitated nursing home residents. Int Psychogeriatr 1:153–165, 1989c

Costa PT, McCrae RR: The NEO-Personality Inventory Manual. Odessa, FL, Psychological Assessment Resources, 1985

Costa PT, McCrae RR: Personality in adulthood: a six-year longitudinal study of self-reports and spouse ratings on the NEO Personality Inventory. J Pers Soc Psychol 54:853–863, 1988

Deutsch LH, Bylsma FW, Rovner BW, et al: Psychosis and physical aggression in probable Alzheimer's disease. Am J Psychiatry 148:1159–1163, 1991

Devanand DP, Miller L, Richard SM, et al: The Columbia University Scale for Psychopathology in Alzheimer's Disease. Arch Neurol 49:371–376, 1992

Eisdorfer C, Cohen D, Paveza GJ, et al: An empirical evaluation of the global deterioration scale for staging Alzheimer's disease. Am J Psychiatry 149:190–194, 1992

Finkel SI, Lyons JS, Anderson RL: Reliability and validity of the Cohen-Mansfield Agitation Inventory in institutionalized elderly. International Journal of Geriatric Psychiatry 7:487–490, 1992

Finkel SI, Lyons JS, Anderson RL: A Brief Agitation Rating Scale (BARS) for nursing home elderly. J Am Geriatr Soc 41:50–52, 1993

Fisher AG: Development of a functional assessment that adjusts ability measures for task simplicity and rater leniency, in Objective Measurement—Theory into Practice. Edited by Wilson M. Norwood, NJ, Ablex, 1994, pp 145–175

Folstein MF, Folstein SE, McHugh PR: "Mini-Mental State": a practical method for grading the cognitive state of patients for the clinician. J Psychiatr Res 12:189–198, 1975

Giordani B, Boivin MJ, Hall AL, et al: The utility and generality of Mini-Mental State Examination scores in Alzheimer's disease. Neurology 40:1894–1896, 1990

Helmes E: Multidimensional Observation Scale for Elderly Subjects (MOSES). Psychopharmacol Bull 24:733–745, 1988

Helmes E, Csapo KG, Short JA: Standardization and validation of the Multidemensional Observation Scale for Elderly Subjects (MOSES). J Gerontol 42:395–405, 1987

Hughes CP, Berg L, Danziger WL, et al: A new clinical scale for the staging of dementia. Br J Psychiatry 140:566–572, 1982

Kane RA, Kane RL: Assessing the Elderly. Lexington, MA, DC Heath, 1981, pp 39–67

Katona CLE, Aldridge CR: The dexamethasone suppression test and depressive signs in dementia. J Affect Disord 8:83–89, 1985

Levin HS, High WM, Goethe KE, et al: The Neurobehavioral Rating Scale Assessment of the behavioral sequelae of head injury by the clinician. J Neurol Neurosurg Psychiatry 50:183–193, 1987

Loewenstein DA, Amigo E, Duara R, et al: A new scale for the assessment of functional status in Alzheimer's disease and related disorders. J Gerontol 44:114–121, 1989

Lukovits TG, McDaniel KD: Behavioral disturbance in severe Alzheimer's disease: a comparison of family member and nursing staff reporting. J Am Geriatr Soc 40:891–895, 1992

Mungas D, Weiler P, Franzi C, et al: Assessment of disruptive behavior associated with dementia: the Disruptive Behavior Rating Scales. J Geriatr Psychiatry Neurol 2:196–202, 1989

Naugle RI, Kawczak K: Limitations of the Mini-Mental State Examination. Cleve Clinic J Med 56:277–281, 1989

Oakley F, Sunderland T, Hill JL, et al: The Daily Activities Questionnaire: a functional assessment for people with Alzheimer's disease. Physical and Occupational Therapy in Geriatrics 10:67–81, 1991

Overall JE, Beller SA: The Brief Psychiatric Rating Scale (BPRS) in geropsychiatric research, I: factor structure on an inpatient unit. J Gerontol 39:187–193, 1984

Overall JE, Gorham DR: The Brief Psychiatric Rating Scale. Psychol Rep 10:799–812, 1962

Overall JE, Rhoades HM: Clinician-rated scales for multidimensional assessment of psychopathology in the elderly. Psychopharmacol Bull 24:587–594, 1988

Petry S, Cummings JL, Hill MA, et al: Personality alterations in dementia of the Alzheimer type. Arch Neurol 45:1187–1190, 1988

Petry S, Cummings JL, Hill MA, et al: Personality alterations in dementia of the Alzheimer type: a three-year follow-up study. J Geriatr Psychiatry Neurol 2:203–207, 1989

Raskin A, Crook T: Relative's Assessment of Global Symptomatology. Psychopharmacol Bull 24:759–763, 1988

Reed BR, Jagust WJ, Seab JP: Mental status as a predictor of daily function in progressive dementia. Gerontologist 29:804–807, 1989

Reisberg B, Ferris SH: A clinical rating scale for symptoms of psychosis in Alzheimer's disease. Psychopharmacol Bull 21:101–104, 1985

Reisberg B, Ferris SH, DeLeon MJ, et al: The Global Deterioration Scale for Assessment of Primary Degenerative Dementia. Am J Psychiatry 139:1136–1139, 1982

Reisberg B, Franssen E, Sclan SG, et al: BEHAVE-AD: A clinical rating scale for the assessment of pharmacologically remediable behavioral symptomatology in Alzheimer's disease, in Alzheimer's Disease: Problems, Prospects, and Perspectives. Edited by Altman HJ. New York, Plenum, 1987a, pp 1–16

Reisberg B, Borenstein J, Salob SP, et al: Behavioral symptoms in Alzheimer's disease: phenomenology and treatment. J Clin Psychiatry 48 (suppl 5):9–15, 1987b

Reisberg B, Ferris SH, DeLeon MJ, et al: Global Deterioration Scale (GDS). Psychopharmacol Bull 24:661–663, 1988

Reisberg B, Franssen E, Sclan S: Stage-specific incidence of potentially remediable behavioral symptoms in aging and Alzheimer's disease—a study of 120 patients using the BEHAVE-AD. Bull Clin Neurosci 54:95–112, 1989

Rosen WG, Mohs RC, Davis KL: A new rating scale for Alzheimer's disease. Am J Psychiatry 141:1356–1364, 1984

Satlin A, Teicher MH, Lieberman HR, et al: Circadian locomotor activity rhythms in Alzheimer's disease. Neuropsychopharmacology 5:115–126, 1991

Saxton J, Swihart AA: Neuropsychological assessment of the severely impaired elderly patient. New Developments in Neuropsychological Evaluation 5:531–543, 1989

Schultz SC, Pato CN (eds): Examples of assessment instruments for use with the aged. Psychopharmacol Bull 24:627–688, 1988

Schwartz GE: Development and validation of the Geriatric Evaluation by Relative's Rating Instrument (GERRI). Psychol Rep 53:479–488, 1983

Schwartz GE: Geriatric Evaluation by Relative's Rating Instrument (GERRI). Psychopharmacol Bull 24:713–716, 1988

Seigler IC, Welsh KA, Dawson DV: Ratings of personality change in patients being evaluated for memory disorders. Alzheimer Dis Assoc Disord 5:240–250, 1991

Shader RI, Harmatz JS, Salzman C: A new scale for clinical assessment in geriatric populations: Sandoz Clinical Assessment—Geriatric (SCAG). J Am Geriatr Soc 22:107–113, 1974

Shader RI, Harmatz JS, Salzman C: Sandoz Clinical Assessment—Geriatric (SCAG). Psychopharmacol Bull 24:765–769, 1988

Sinha D, Zemlan FP, Nelson S, et al: A new scale for assessing behavioral agitation in dementia. Psychiatry Res 41:73–88, 1992

Skurla E, Rogers JC, Sunderland T: Direct assessment of activities of daily living in Alzheimer's disease. J Am Geriatr Soc 36:97–103, 1988

Spinnler H, DellaSala S: The role of clinical neuropsychology in the neurological diagnosis of Alzheimer's disease. J Neurol 235:258–271, 1988

Sultzer DL, Levin HS, Mahler ME, et al: Assessment of cognitive, psychiatric, and behavioral disturbances in patients with dementia: the Neurobehavioral Rating Scale. J Am Geriatr Soc 40:549–555, 1992

Sunderland T, Alterman IS, Yount D, et al: A new scale for the assessment of depressed mood in dementia subjects. Am J Psychiatry 145:955–959, 1988

Tariot PN, Mack JL, Patterson MB, et al: CERAD Behavior Rating Scale for Dementia. Am J Psychiatry (in press)

Teicher MH, Lawrence JM, Barber NI, et al: Altered locomotor activity in neuropsychiatric patients. Prog Neuropsychopharmacol Biol Psychiatry 10:755–761, 1986

Teri L, Larson EB, Reifler BV: Behavioral disturbance in dementia of the Alzheimer's type. J Am Geriatr Soc 36:1–6, 1988

Teri L, Borson S, Kiyaket HA, et al: Behavioral disturbance, cognitive dysfunction, and functional skill-prevalence and relationship in Alzheimer's disease. J Am Geriatr Soc 37:109–116, 1989

Teri L, Truax P, Logsdon R, et al: Assessment of behavioral problems in dementia: the Revised Memory and Behavior Problems Checklist. Psychol Aging 7:622–631, 1992

Section III

Management Strategies

CHAPTER 7

Role of Neuroleptics in Treatment of Behavioral Complications

D. P. Devanand, M.D.

*I*n recent years, increased attention has been paid to the phenomenology and treatment of behavioral complications in Alzheimer's disease (Devanand et al. 1989; Reisberg et al. 1987; Schneider et al. 1990). This focus is partly due to the recognition that behavioral problems and psychosis develop in a large number of Alzheimer's disease patients at some point during the course of the illness and also due to the expectation that such symptoms can be treated successfully with medications, unlike the cognitive deficits of Alzheimer's disease. In this chapter the term *behavioral complications* encompasses both behavioral disturbances (e.g., apathy, agitation, wandering) and psychotic features (e.g., delusions and hallucinations).

Behavioral complications occur frequently in Alzheimer's disease (Reisberg et al. 1987; Seltzer and Sherwin 1983), include a wide variety of symptoms (Devanand et al. 1992a; Rabins et al. 1982), and are distressing to patients and caregivers. Even modest improvement in behavioral symptoms may result in substantial

---

Supported in part by Grant MH44176 from the National Institute of Mental Health.

improvement in functioning and quality of life (Shulman and Steinberg 1984), whereas untreated behavioral problems may lead to institutionalization (Haller et al. 1989). The most common use of drugs in dementia, including Alzheimer's disease, is in the management of behavioral disturbance, and almost every patient with dementia will receive at least one psychoactive agent during the course of illness (Terry and Katzman 1983). In this chapter, I review the extant research on the use of neuroleptics in Alzheimer's disease.

Neuroleptics in the Treatment of Behavioral Complications

Based largely on the evidence that neuroleptics are efficacious in the treatment of a variety of psychotic disorders, the presumption has been that if delusions and hallucinations are present, neuroleptics are likely to be effective regardless of diagnosis (Raskind and Risse 1986). It has also been suggested that neuroleptics may be effective in the treatment of bizarre and disturbing behaviors in Alzheimer's disease that cannot be understood in terms of impaired memory or aphasia (Raskind and Risse 1986), although making this distinction is often difficult, particularly when the patient's ability to communicate diminishes with disease progression (Devanand et al. 1988).

Neuroleptics tend to be used in Alzheimer's disease when delusions and hallucinations, often of a paranoid nature, complicate the course of dementia (Raskind and Risse 1986). However, classic psychotic symptoms such as delusions and hallucinations are less common than behavioral problems such as agitation and catastrophic reactions in Alzheimer's disease (Devanand et al. 1992a, 1992b). Thus the presentation of these nonpsychotic behavioral symptoms, particularly agitation, more commonly leads to treatment with neuroleptics. Some studies suggested that classic psychotic symptoms may be more responsive to neuroleptics than are other behavioral disturbances (Devanand et al. 1989; Petrie et al. 1982), but to clarify this issue, further systematic research is required. Another poorly studied question is whether some delusions that are clearly secondary to cognitive impairment—for example, the belief that deceased parents are alive—are less likely to respond to neuroleptics (Raskind and Risse 1986).

Prevalence of Neuroleptic Usage

In a survey of 1,276 geriatric inpatients at 12 Veterans Administration hospitals, 61% were receiving psychoactive drugs (Prien et al. 1975). Of patients with organic brain syndrome, 55% were receiving drugs, and the most frequently prescribed agents were neuroleptics (44%), followed by antidepressants (11%) and antianxiety agents (10%). Patients over age 75 received less than half the dose administered to patients aged 60–65, and the latter received an average of 229 mg of chlorpromazine equivalents daily. Another study of 101 inpatients with dementia found that 38 received one psychotropic agent and 20 received two; neuroleptics were most commonly used (Michel and Kolakowska 1981). In 839 institutionalized geriatric patients in a London borough, neuroleptic usage ranged from 0 to 44% in different wards (Gilleard et al. 1983). In studies conducted in the United States, nursing home usage of psychotropic medications appears to vary considerably, ranging from 11% (Reynolds 1984) to 74% (Ray et al. 1980) in different studies. More recent studies indicate that the high prevalence of psychotropic medication usage in long-term care facilities has not changed (Avorn et al. 1989; Beardsley et al. 1989; Beers et al. 1988; Lantz et al. 1990). Neuroleptics and benzodiazepines are the agents used most frequently, and psychotropic medications are often combined with other centrally acting agents.

Psychotropic medications have been used commonly in nursing homes for at least two decades (Barton and Hurst 1966), and this practice has led to an outcry of disapproval by some of the media in the United States. However, it remains unclear how many of these nursing home patients are receiving neuroleptics unnecessarily, and the efficacy of alternative pharmacological or behavioral approaches to managing behavioral complications in Alzheimer's disease remains to be established (Schneider and Sobin 1991). In outpatients, the prevalence of neuroleptic usage appears to be lower (Devanand et al. 1992a; Reisberg et al. 1987; Wragg and Jeste 1989).

In clinical practice, it is often possible to taper or withdraw neuroleptics over time, presumably because some Alzheimer's disease patients experience a remission of behavioral complications that is due to pathological changes in specific brain regions that accompany illness progression. Limited indirect evidence supports this view. Lantz et al. (1990), in a study of 91 nursing home patients of whom half had dementia, found that more than half of the 91 had received a psychotropic medication during their 5 years of residence, but that less than a fourth of the 91 were continuously medicated.

Uncontrolled Studies of Neuroleptics in Dementia

Most studies of neuroleptics in dementia, both controlled and uncontrolled, have been of relatively short duration (3–8 weeks on average). Several early uncontrolled studies evaluated the efficacy and side effects of neuroleptics in geriatric patients in hospitals or nursing homes. Many of these studies were of diagnostically heterogeneous samples, and they often included patients with other primary disorders such as schizophrenia or major affective disorders that are known to be responsive to treatment (Branchey et al. 1978; Cavero 1966; Jackson 1961; Kral 1961; Robinson 1959; Tewfik et al. 1970; Tobin et al. 1970). Studies of samples of patients of whom most had dementia also tended to be diagnostically heterogeneous (Terman 1955; Tobin et al. 1970), and few restricted the inclusion criteria to Alzheimer's disease only (Gottlieb et al. 1988; Steele et al. 1986; Tune et al. 1991). These uncontrolled investigations suggested that between 25% and 75% of the patients showed improvement in behavioral symptomatology (Reisberg et al. 1987; Kral 1961), whereas other studies were equivocal or negative about the efficacy of neuroleptics for behavioral disturbance over a diagnostically broad spectrum (Goldstein and Dippy 1967; Robinson 1959; Tewfik et al. 1970). Traditional side effects of neuroleptics were described in several of these studies, but there is little information on the effects of neuroleptics on cognition or activities of daily life in Alzheimer's disease (Lehmann and Ban 1967; Steele et al. 1986).

Controlled Studies of Neuroleptics in Dementia

Early studies comparing chlorpromazine with placebo in samples restricted to organic mental disorders failed to demonstrate significantly superior efficacy for neuroleptics (Abse et al. 1960; Barton and Hurst 1966). In a more recent study, Coccaro et al. (1990) conducted an 8-week trial in a group of 52 elderly residents of long-term care facilities who were randomized to one of three medications: haloperidol ($n = 18$), oxazepam ($n = 17$), and diphenhydramine ($n = 17$). The authors found low doses of all three to be modestly efficacious, with few side effects. The absence of a parallel-group placebo condition is a major design limitation of this study. In fact, few of the studies in which dementia patients formed a majority of the sample used a randomized, double-blind, placebo-controlled design (Table 7–1). Some of these controlled studies found evidence of moderate efficacy for neuroleptics in the treatment of behavioral complications. The inconsistencies noted between studies may partly be accounted for by the placebo response rate, which varied from 9% to 50% across studies (Table 7–1). Several additional limitations of these reports were described in several other reviews (Devanand et al. 1988; Salzman 1987; Schneider et al. 1990; Sunderland and Silver 1988): 1) diagnostic heterogeneity was a frequent feature in patient samples, 2) methods of assessment were often global and inadequate, 3) the effects of neuroleptics on core psychotic features versus other forms of behavioral disturbances were not distinguished from each other, and 4) virtually all the studies were conducted with inpatients who probably had severe dementia.

During the last two decades, only three random-assignment, double-blind, placebo-controlled trials of neuroleptics have been conducted in dementia patients who were either inpatients or residents of nursing homes (Table 7–1). Rada and Kellner (1976) conducted a 4-week trial in 42 patients (mean age 75.5 years) with

Table 7–1. Randomized double-blind placebo-controlled studies of neuroleptics in samples of patients, majority with dementia

Report	N	Diagnosis	Length (wks)	Medication and mg/day	Outcome measures	Results
Abse et al. 1960	32	OBS + senile psychosis	8	Chlorpromazine 75	Global; target symptoms	Improvement on drug and placebo
Hamilton and Bennett 1962a	19	OBS with psychosis	3–8	Acetophenazine 40	Behavior; nursing scales	Worse on medication
Hamilton and Bennett 1962b	27	OBS with psychosis 78%	8	Trifluperazine 4–8	Behavior; nursing scales	Worse on medication
Sugarman et al. 1964	18	OBS	6	Haloperidol 0.5–4.5; benztropine prn	Psychotic reaction profile	Agitation and hostility improved
Rada and Kellner 1976	42	Nonpsychotic OBS 57%; psychotic OBS 43%	4	Thiothixene 6–15	BPRS; NOSIE	Ineffective but safe
Barnes et al. 1982	53	PDD 55%; MID 38%, other 7%	8	Thioridazine 62.5; loxapine 10.5	BPRS; SCAG; CGI; NOSIE	All groups improved on BPRS
Petrie et al. 1982	61	PDD 49%; MID 43%, other 8%	8	Haloperidol 4.6; loxapine 21.9	BPRS; SCAG; CGI	Some improvement: 35% haloperidol; 32% loxapine; 9% placebo

Note. OBS, organic brain syndrome. MID, multi-infarct dementia. PDD, primary degenerative dementia. BPRS, Brief Psychiatric Rating Scale. SCAG, Sandoz Clinical Assessment—Geriatric. CGI, Clinical Global Improvement. NOSIE, Nurses Observation Scale for Inpatient Evaluation.

organic brain syndrome (by DSM-II criteria), of whom 24 had the nonpsychotic form and 18 had the psychotic form. The only significant difference between thiothixene (n = 22, up to 15 mg/day) and placebo (n = 20) was on the Manifest Psychosis factor on the Nurses Observation Scale for Inpatient Evaluation, in favor of thiothixene. Adverse effects were minimal in both groups. The report lacked information on comparability between groups with respect to psychosis, and what proportion of patients would meet current criteria for Alzheimer's disease remains unclear. Further, the very high placebo response rate (55%) and the short trial duration are problematic.

Petrie et al. (1982) studied 61 dementia patients (mean age 73 years) of whom 30 (49%) had primary degenerative dementia and 26 (43%) had multi-infarct dementia. Patients were randomized to loxapine, haloperidol, or placebo (Table 7–1). Moderate or marked global clinical improvement occurred in 35% of the haloperidol group, 32% of the loxapine group, and 9% of the placebo group. The two drug-treated groups showed significant improvement on specific items and total scores on the Brief Psychiatric Rating Scale (BPRS) and the Sandoz Clinical Assessment—Geriatric (SCAG). Adverse effects were noted in 90% of both the loxapine and the haloperidol groups and in 55% of the placebo group, but further details were not given. There are several limitations in applying the results to guide the clinician: 1) the large proportion of patients with multi-infarct dementia (42.6%), 2) the use of antiparkinsonian agents and chloral hydrate as needed, and 3) the relatively high dose of haloperidol (mean 4.6 mg daily), which may have increased the likelihood of side effects.

Barnes et al. (1982) studied 53 patients (mean age 83 years) with a DSM-III diagnosis of dementia who were randomized to thioridazine, loxapine, or placebo (Table 7–1). All groups improved from baseline on the BPRS, and there was only a modest advantage for the two neuroleptics. Loxapine was significantly superior to placebo in treating anxiety, excitement, emotional lability, and uncooperativeness. Adverse effects were reported in 33% of the thioridazine group, 45% of the loxapine group, and 16% of the placebo group. The high rate of clinical response in the placebo group raises questions about sample selection in this study. Another important confound is the concomitant use of trihexyphenidyl and chloral hydrate as needed (Barnes et al. 1982).

In summary, even the three most rigorous, widely quoted controlled studies of neuroleptics in dementia suffered from serious methodological flaws (Devanand et al. 1988; Salzman 1987; Schneider et al. 1990; Sunderland and Silver 1988). There has been no published randomized, double-blind, placebo-controlled study of neuroleptics to treat behavioral complications in a sample restricted to Alzheimer's disease patients in which concomitant psychotropic medications were not allowed. Schneider et al. (1990) conducted a metanalysis of published placebo-controlled trials of neuroleptics in agitated dementia patients, evaluating all studies that included patients with any form of organic brain syndrome. Studies involving this broad spectrum of patients were chosen presumably because of the lack of extant data on samples restricted to a single diagnosis such as Alzheimer's disease. The metanalysis revealed a modest effect for neuroleptics compared with placebo (one-tailed $P = .004$) and a small effect size ($r = .18$), indicating that 18% of dementia patients benefited from neuroleptic treatment beyond that of placebo. As the authors noted, clinical worsening, noncompleters, and the impact of treatment-emergent effects could not be accounted for in the metanalysis. The studies reviewed were inpatient studies, and it is unclear whether similar findings will be obtained in outpatient studies, where few controlled data are available (Devanand et al. 1989).

The problem of diagnostic heterogeneity in sample selection and other major methodological limitations that characterize virtually all the studies in this area severely limit the utility of metanalytic techniques. Further, sample selection is a critical factor that metanalysis cannot take into account adequately. Another major concern is that two of the three major studies conducted in the last two decades demonstrated a high placebo response rate (Barnes et al. 1982; Rada and Kellner 1976), with the implication that patients with very mild behavioral changes may have been included for the purpose of increasing sample size. Patients of this type are unlikely to demonstrate a drug-placebo difference. The inclusion of mildly disturbed patients in studies is particularly problematic in Alzheimer's disease, in which mild behavioral changes are far more common than severe behavioral complications and may be of insufficient severity to merit intervention with neuroleptics (Devanand et al. 1992a, 1992b). Inclusion of these patients in several research studies may have resulted in the spurious finding of lack of efficacy for neuroleptics (Type II error).

Comparisons Between Neuroleptics

Among neuroleptics, thioridazine may be the most frequently prescribed drug (Lantz et al. 1990). Studies that compared a low-potency neuroleptic, thioridazine, with a high-potency neuroleptic, haloperidol, did not demonstrate any consistent differences in efficacy (Cowley and Glen 1979; Rosen 1979; Smith et al. 1974; Tsuang et al. 1971). These studies were limited by the lack of a placebo control and by the fact that the patient samples were diagnostically heterogeneous. Unfortunately, little work has been done on the effects of neuroleptics on cognition and activities of daily life in Alzheimer's disease (Devanand et al. 1989). It thus remains unclear whether the anticholinergic effects of thioridazine negatively affect cognitive function to a greater extent than do the anticholinergic effects of high-potency neuroleptics (e.g., haloperidol) that have relatively low anticholinergic profiles. Overall, there is little evidence to favor one neuroleptic over another in terms of efficacy, judging from studies that have compared thioridazine with another neuroleptic and a few studies that have compared haloperidol with another neuroleptic (Salzman 1987). The choice of neuroleptic should be based on side effect profiles rather than expectations of differential efficacy.

Studies Comparing Neuroleptics to Other Agents

In dementia patients with behavioral complications, comparisons between neuroleptics and other psychotropic agents have been restricted primarily to benzodiazepines. A recent study of 21 behaviorally disturbed dementia inpatients on a psychogeriatric unit revealed no significant differences between the group receiving haloperidol (0.5–3 mg daily) and the one receiving oxazepam (10–30 mg daily); both groups showed modest decreases in targeted aberrant behaviors (Burgio et al. 1992). Prior studies comparing benzodiazepines with neuroleptics in the management of nonpsychotic behaviorally disturbed dementia patients have been inconclusive. Tewfik et al. (1970) claimed superiority for oxazepam compared with several neuroleptics in a study involving diagnostically heterogeneous geriatric patients, whereas other studies demonstrated superiority for thioridazine over benzodiazepines in the treatment of anxiety and agitation in nursing homes and similar facilities (Covington 1975; Kirven and Montero 1973; Stotsky 1984). Despite the established findings that benzodiazepines can have deleterious effects on learning and memory in cognitively normal subjects (Ghoneim et al. 1981; Jones et al. 1978; Liljequist et al. 1978), particularly among elderly people (Pomara et al. 1990), side effect comparisons of neuroleptics and benzodiazepines in Alzheimer's disease have not been reported.

There are major methodological limitations to all these studies, with respect to both sample selection and study design. These limited data do not support the view that benzodiazepines are superior to neuroleptics in the treatment of behavioral problems in nonpsychotic patients with dementia.

Side Effects and Interactions With Other Drugs

Neuroleptic drugs undergo biotransformation primarily in the liver; the gastrointestinal tract, the lungs, and the kidneys are less important sites. On average, drugs have slightly longer medication half-lives in elderly people compared with the rest of the population (Davis 1981; Hicks and Davis 1980). Elderly patients tend to be prone to adverse effects of drugs because of their decreased tolerance and a narrowing of the therapeutic index of these drugs (Baldessarini 1985). Age-related decreases in gut motility and the anticholinergic effects of neuroleptics may slow gastric emptying, thereby decreasing the rate of absorption. Therefore, although it may take longer for the drugs to reach therapeutic levels in the blood, it may also take longer for the drugs to leave the system, and side effects may thereby be prolonged. This type of effect was observed in a preliminary study using haloperidol in doses of 1–4 mg daily in Alzheimer's disease (Devanand et al. 1989).

Antacids, commonly used in elderly people, may lower neuroleptic levels (Fann et al. 1973; Forrest et al. 1970).

Largely because of the physiological changes that occur with aging, neuroleptic medications are more difficult to use in elderly patients than in younger patients. There is an increased propensity to side effects, both short-term and long-term (Devanand et al. 1988; Harris et al. 1992; Prien 1973; Raskind and Risse 1986). This increase in side effects in elderly patients occurs in the areas of anticholinergic side effects, extrapyramidal side effects, and the likelihood of developing tardive dyskinesia (Glazer and Morgenstern 1988; Tepper and Haas 1979; Wragg and Jeste 1988). As a result, elderly schizophrenic patients tend to be maintained on neuroleptic doses that are one-third to one-half those used in young adults (Prien 1973). In Alzheimer's disease it appears that even lower doses should be used, because not only are there physiological changes due to aging, but the direct destruction of brain neurons with disease progression renders Alzheimer's disease patients particularly vulnerable to central nervous system side effects, primarily extrapyramidal ones (Devanand et al. 1989). However, there is little information about how long an Alzheimer's disease patient should be continued on neuroleptics or about their side effect profile with chronic use in Alzheimer's disease, including the risk of developing tardive dyskinesia. In a series of 14 patients with Alzheimer's disease confirmed by autopsy, McDaniel et al. (1991) reported that 4 patients with clinical evidence of tardive dyskinesia showed greater degenerative changes in the substantia nigra than 10 patients without evidence of tardive dyskinesia.

Other complications of neuroleptics include neuroleptic malignant syndrome and cardiac side effects, including orthostatic hypotension with low-potency neuroleptics (Blumenthal and Davie 1980). Less common side effects include hepatotoxicity (chlorpromazine), retinopathy (thioridazine), agranulocytosis, dermatological reactions, arrhythmias, and even sudden death.

The side effect profile often determines the choice of neuro-leptic—for example, the Alzheimer's disease patient with base-line hypotension may receive haloperidol, whereas thioridazine may be preferred in the Alzheimer's disease patient with preex-isting parkinsonian signs. Given the increased risk of cardiovas-cular side effects and the anticholinergic symptoms of confusion, urinary retention, and constipation in elderly patients, haloperi-dol may be the medically safer choice in many cases. These factors need to be weighed against the greatly increased sensitiv-ity to extrapyramidal side effects in Alzheimer's disease, particu-larly with high-potency drugs such as haloperidol (Devanand et al. 1989; Tune et al. 1991). Further, elderly people often take many medications, increasing the risk of significant drug interactions (Salzman 1982).

Petrie et al. (1982) calculated that neuroleptics (haloperidol or loxapine) caused sedation in 38% of their patients and caused extrapyramidal side effects in 38%. The doses used (mean halo-peridol 4.6 mg daily and loxapine 21.9 mg daily) were somewhat higher than those currently recommended for use in Alzheimer's disease (Devanand et al. 1989; Tune et al. 1991). In a single-blind, placebo-controlled pilot study of nine Alzheimer's disease pa-tients with behavioral complications, we found that oral halo-peridol in doses of 1–5 mg daily was effective in treating behavioral complications (Devanand et al. 1989). However, side effects, particularly extrapyramidal signs, tended to be severe at higher doses, and no patient could be maintained on more than 4 mg of haloperidol daily. Scores on a modified Mini-Mental State Exam (MMSE) worsened on haloperidol, suggesting that in Alz-heimer's disease patients the effects of neuroleptics on cognition, in addition to traditional neuroleptic side effects, need to be evaluated during the course of clinical management. Risse et al. (1987) described two agitated Alzheimer's disease patients who either worsened or did not respond to conventional low-dose neuroleptic treatment but demonstrated sustained improvement with very low dose treatment (haloperidol 0.125 mg daily for one patient and thioridazine 5 mg daily for the other).

In another pilot study of 10 Alzheimer's disease patients, depot neuroleptic treatment with low-dose fluphenazine deca-noate (1.25–3.75 mg im bimonthly) was efficacious, with few side effects observed during a 16-week trial (Gottlieb et al. 1988). In an open trial of 30 Alzheimer's disease patients with behavioral problems who received low-dose haloperidol (0.5–3 mg daily) or thioridazine (12.5–75 mg daily), Tune et al. (1991) found that most patients developed side effects and only 3 completed the study without experiencing significant side effects. During a 3-month stabilization follow-up phase, late-emerging side effects developed in 7 of 18 patients. It remains unclear whether these side effects are purely a function of neuroleptic use or are a function of the progression of Alzheimer's disease pathology in the brain. Although limited by the open-trial design, the findings by Tune et al. (1991) support the view that both short-term and longer-term side effects are frequent limiting factors during neuroleptic usage in Alzheimer's disease, even when low doses are used.

Effects on Cognition and Activities of Daily Life

There is no evidence that neuroleptics directly ameliorate the cognitive dysfunction of dementia, and there is some preliminary evidence that haloperidol in doses of more than 4 mg/day results in significant worsening of cognitive function, as assessed by scores on a modified MMSE (Devanand et al. 1989). Although haloperidol is a drug with relatively low anticholinergic effects, it is possible that this anticholinergic activity may further compromise the already impaired central cholinergic systems in patients with Alzheimer's disease (Davies and Maloney 1976; Perry et al. 1977). The level of cognitive impairment in Alzheimer's disease may be worsened by the use of neuroleptics with strong anticholinergic properties (e.g., thioridazine) or by the use of additional anticholinergic agents used to control drug-induced parkinsonian symptoms. Another possibility is that the sedation produced by neuroleptics enhances the level of disorientation and cognitive impairment in Alzheimer's disease. These theoretical considerations remain to be validated by systematic clinical trials, and further work is needed to evaluate the impact of neuroleptics on cognition and the ability to perform the activities of daily life.

Blood Levels

Little work has examined the utility of monitoring neuroleptic blood levels in Alzheimer's disease. We recently found that an oral dose of haloperidol correlated very strongly with blood levels in 19 Alzheimer's disease patients (r = .82, P = .0001) (Devanand et al. 1992c). We hypothesized that the absence of prior exposure to neuroleptics in these Alzheimer's disease patients may have precluded the alterations in drug absorption and metabolism that are known to occur in schizophrenia, with resultant distortion of the relationship between oral dose and blood level. Therapeutic effects were observed in these Alzheimer's disease patients at blood levels that in most cases were below the postulated "therapeutic window" of 4–18 ng/ml for haloperidol blood levels in schizophrenia (Mavroidis et al. 1985; Volavka and Cooper 1987). Further, compared with oral dose, blood levels showed stronger associations with changes in symptoms and changes in severity of extrapyramidal side effects (Devanand et al. 1992c). Although intriguing, these preliminary findings on the utility of monitoring neuroleptic blood levels require further extension and independent replication.

Optimum Neuroleptic Dosage

Given the problem of side effects at conventional low doses of neuroleptics in Alzheimer's disease, the question of whether homeopathic doses will maintain efficacy, while reducing side effects, remains to be answered. In our current state of knowledge, the equivalent of 0.5–1 mg of haloperidol daily should be the starting dose in Alzheimer's disease, with subsequent upward or downward dose titration based on clinical response and observed side effects. Ongoing research is likely to define further the dosage at which the optimal tradeoff between efficacy and side effects is obtained.

Guidelines for Clinical Practice

The paucity of controlled studies that employed rigorous methodology limits the strength of any recommendations that can be made to guide clinical practice. The following issues need to be taken into account when neuroleptics are considered for the treatment of behavioral complications in Alzheimer's disease patients:

1. Neuroleptics are more difficult to use in elderly patients compared with younger ones, and this difficulty is increased further with the diagnosis of Alzheimer's disease.
2. Evaluation of the tradeoff between efficacy and side effects is particularly important in Alzheimer's disease, and dosage often needs to be individualized.
3. There is no clear evidence that one neuroleptic is better than any other in treating the behavioral complications of Alzheimer's disease. The choice of medication depends more on the likely side effects than on differential efficacy. If one neuroleptic proves to be ineffective or cannot be tolerated, a trial of an alternative neuroleptic with a different potency and side effect profile may be considered.
4. Neuroleptics may be particularly helpful in Alzheimer's disease patients with paranoid or other delusions or hallucinations and with behavioral problems such as severe agitation.
5. In some cases, neuroleptics can be useful in the treatment of behavioral dyscontrol, hostility, aggression, and perhaps violence in Alzheimer's disease. Patients who are most behaviorally disturbed may show the greatest benefit from treatment, whereas patients with unclear target symptoms that might be caused primarily by the degree of cognitive impairment may be unresponsive. Therefore, neuroleptics must be used only for clearly defined symptomatology.
6. Depending on the prior medical status of the patient, cardiac, renal, and hepatic function may need to be assessed. The risk of interactions with medications that the patient may receive for other conditions needs to be evaluated when neuroleptics are prescribed.
7. The starting dose should be low and titrated gradually upward until there is a clear therapeutic effect or until adverse effects become significant. In most cases, the dosage should be in the range of 0.25–3 mg daily of haloperidol equivalents, because higher doses tend to be associated with severe side

effects, mainly of the extrapyramidal type.

8. Target symptoms should be identified clearly and monitored and assessed serially during treatment.

9. Both traditional neuroleptic side effects (e.g., extrapyramidal signs, akathisia, orthostatic hypotension, and sedation) and the effects on cognition and the activities of daily life should be monitored during neuroleptic therapy in Alzheimer's disease.

10. Anticholinergic agents to treat side effects should be avoided; lowering of the neuroleptic dose is the preferred mode for treating extrapyramidal side effects. If anticholinergics become essential, they should be used sparingly at low dosage.

11. Potential side effects should be discussed before starting drugs. This will often involve the family member.

12. Both the dosage and the duration of therapy should be minimized to the extent possible. Because of the increased risk of tardive dyskinesia in elderly people, periodic attempts should be made to taper or discontinue the drug, although the ideal minimum (or maximum) period of neuroleptic treatment remains to be established. Because the typical duration of episode of behavioral complications in Alzheimer's disease has not been well studied, it remains unclear when exactly the attempt should be made to taper or discontinue effective neuroleptic treatment—for example, 3–6 months after clinical response is obtained.

References

Abse DW, Dahlstrom WG, Hill C: The value of chemotherapy in senile mental disturbance. JAMA 174:2036–2042, 1960

Avorn J, Dreyer P, Connelly K, et al: Use of psychotropic medication and the quality of care in rest homes. N Engl J Med 320:227–232, 1989

Baldessarini RF: Clinical and epidemiologic aspects of tardive dyskinesia. J Clin Psychiatry 46:8–13, 1985

Barnes R, Veith R, Okimoto J, et al: Efficacy of antipsychotic medications in behaviorally disturbed dementia patients. Am J Psychiatry 139:1170–1174, 1982

Barton R, Hurst L: Unnecessary use of tranquilizers in elderly patients. Br J Psychiatry 112:989–990, 1966

Beardsley RS, Larson DB, Burns BJ, et al: Prescribing of psychotropics in elderly nursing home patients. J Am Geriatr Soc 37:327–330, 1989

Beers M, Avorn J, Soumerai SB, et al: Psychoactive medication use in intermediate-care facility residents. JAMA 260:3016–3020, 1988

Blumenthal MD, Davie JW: Dizziness and falling in elderly psychiatric outpatients. Am J Psychiatry 137:203–206, 1980

Branchey MH, Lee JH, Amin R, et al: High- and low-potency neuroleptics in elderly psychiatric patients. JAMA 239:1860–1862, 1978

Burgio LD, Reynolds CFI, Janosky JE, et al: A behavioral microanalysis of the effects of haloperidol and oxazepam in demented psychogeriatric inpatients. International Journal of Geriatric Psychiatry 7:253–262, 1992

Cavero CV: Evaluation of thioridazine in the aged. J Am Geriatr Soc 14:617–622, 1966

Coccaro EF, Kramer E, Zemishlany Z, et al: Pharmacologic treatment of noncognitive behavioral disturbances in elderly demented patients. Am J Psychiatry 147:1640–1645, 1990

Covington JS: Alleviating agitation, apprehension, and related symptoms in geriatric patients. South Med J 58:719–724, 1975

Cowley LM, Glen RS: Double-blind study of thioridazine and haloperidol in geriatric patients with a psychosis associated with organic brain syndrome. J Clin Psychiatry 40:411–419, 1979

Davies P, Maloney AJF: Selective loss of central cholinergic neurons in Alzheimer's disease (letter to the editor). Lancet 1:1403, 1976

Davis JM: Antipsychotics, in Physicians' Handbook on Psychotherapeutic Drug Use in the Aged. Edited by Crook T, Cohen GD. New Cannan, CT, Mark Powley, 1981, pp 12–25

Devanand DP, Sackeim HA, Mayeux R: Psychosis, behavioral disturbance, and the use of neuroleptics in dementia. Compr Psychiatry 29:387–401, 1988

Devanand D, Sackeim H, Brown R, et al: A pilot study of haloperidol treatment of psychosis and behavioral disturbance in Alzheimer's disease. Arch Neurol 46:854–857, 1989

Devanand DP, Brockington CD, Moody BJ, et al: Behavioral Syndromes in Alzheimer's disease. Int Psychogeriatr 4 (suppl 2):161–184, 1992a

Devanand DP, Miller L, Richards M, et al: The Columbia University Scale for Psychopathology in Alzheimer's disease. Arch Neurol 49:371–376, 1992b

Devanand DP, Cooper T, Sackeim HA, et al: Low-dose oral haloperidol and blood levels in Alzheimer's disease: a preliminary study. Psychopharmacol Bull 28:169–173, 1992c

Fann WE, Davis J, Janowsky D, et al: Chlorpromazine: effects of antacids on its gastrointestinal absorption. J Clin Pharmacol 13:388–390, 1973

Forrest FM, Forrest IS, Serra MT: Modification of chlorpromazine metabolism by some other drugs frequently administered to psychiatric patients. Biol Psychiatry 2:53–58, 1970

Ghoneim NM, Mewaldt SP, Berie JL, et al: Memory and performance effects of single and 3-week administration of diazepam. Psychopharmacology 73:147–151, 1981

Gilleard CJ, Morgan K, Wade BE: Patterns of neuroleptic use among the institutionalized elderly. Acta Psychiatr Scand 68:419–425, 1983

Glazer W, Morgenstern H: Predictors of occurrence, severity and course of tardive dyskinesia in an outpatient population. J Clin Psychopharmacol 8:10S–16S, 1988

Goldstein BJ, Dippy WE: A clinical evaluation of mesoridazine (Serentil) in geriatric patients. Current Therapeutic Research 9:256–260, 1967

Gottlieb GL, McAllister TW, Gur RC: Depot neuroleptics in the treatment of behavioral disorders in patients with Alzheimer's disease. J Am Geriatr Soc 36:642–644, 1988

Hamilton LD, Bennett JL: Acetophenazine for hyperactive geriatric patients. Geriatrics 17:596–601, 1962a

Hamilton LD, Bennett JL: The use of trifluoperazine in geriatric patients with chronic brain syndrome. J Am Geriatr Soc 10:140–147, 1962b

Harris MJ, Panton D, Caligiuri MP, et al: High incidence of tardive dyskinesia in older outpatients on low doses of neuroleptics. Psychopharmacol Bull 28:87–92, 1992

Hicks R, Davis J: Pharmacokinetics in geriatric psychopharmacology, in Psychopharmacology of Aging. Edited by Eisdorfer C, Fann W. New York, Spectrum Publications, 1980, pp 169–212

Jackson EB: Mellaril in the treatment of the geriatric patient. Am J Psychiatry 118:543–544, 1961

Jones DM, Lewis MJ, Spriggs TLB: The effects of low doses of diazepam on human performance in group administered tasks. Br J Clin Pharmacol 6:333–337, 1978

Kirven LG, Montero EF: Comparison of thioridazine and diazepam in the control of nonpsychotic symptoms associated with senility: double-blind study. J Am Geriatr Soc 21:546–551, 1973

Kral VA: The use of thioridazine (Mellaril) in aged people. Can Med Assoc J 84:152–154, 1961

Lantz MS, Louis A, Lowenstein G, et al: A longitudinal study of psychotropic prescriptions in a teaching nursing home. Am J Psychiatry 147:1637–1639, 1990

Liljequist R, Linnoila M, Mattila MJ: Effect of diazepam and chlorpromazine on memory functions in man. Eur J Clin Pharmacol 13:339–343, 1978

Mavroidis ML, Garver DL, Kanter DR, et al: Plasma haloperidol levels and clinical response: confounding variables. Psychopharmacol Bull 21:62–65, 1985

McDaniel KD, Kazee AM, Eskin TA, et al: Tardive dyskinesia in Alzheimer's disease: clinical features and neuropathologic correlates. J Geriatr Psychiatry Neurol 4:79–85, 1991

Michel K, Kolakowska T: A survey of prescribing psychotropic drugs in two psychiatric hospitals. Br J Psychiatry 138:217–221, 1981

Patterson J: A preliminary study of carabamazepine in the treatment of assaultive patients with dementia. J Geriatr Psychiatry Neurol 1:21–23, 1988

Perry EK, Gibson PH, Blessed G, et al: Neurotransmitter enzyme abnormalities in senile dementia. J Neurol Sci 34:247–265, 1977

Petrie WM, Lawson EC, Hollender MH: Violence in geriatric patients. JAMA 248:443–444, 1982

Pomara N, Deptula D, Singh R, et al: Cognitive toxicity of benzodiazepines in the elderly, in Anxiety in the Elderly: Treatment and Research. Edited by Salzman C, Lebowitz B. New York, Springer, 1990, pp 175–196

Prien RF: Chemotherapy in organic brain syndrome: a review of the literature. Psychopharmacol Bull 9:5–20, 1973

Prien Y, Haber PA, Caffey EMJ: The use of psychoactive drugs in elderly patients with psychiatric disorders: survey conducted in twelve Veterans Administration hospitals. J Am Geriatr Soc 23:104–112, 1975

Rada RT, Kellner R: Thiothixene in the treatment of geriatric patients with chronic organic brain syndrome. J Am Geriatr Soc 24:105–107, 1976

Raskind MA, Risse SC: Antipsychotic drugs and the elderly. J Clin Psychiatry 47:17–22, 1986

Ray WA, Federspiel CF, Schaffner W: A study of antipsychotic drug use in nursing homes: epidemiologic evidence suggesting misuse. Am J Public Health 70:485–491, 1980

Reisberg B, Borenstein J, Salob SP, et al: Behavioral symptoms in Alzheimer's disease: phenomenology and treatment. J Clin Psychiatry 48:9–15, 1987

Reynolds MD: Institutional prescribing for the elderly: patterns of prescribing in a municipal hospital and a municipal nursing home. J Am Geriatr Soc 32:640–645, 1984

Risse SC, Lampe TH, Cubberley L: Very low-dose neuroleptic treatment in two patients with agitation associated with Alzheimer's disease. J Clin Psychiatry 48:207–208, 1987

Robinson DB: Evaluation of certain drugs in geriatric patients. Arch Gen Psychiatry 1:41–47, 1959

Rosen JH: Double-blind comparison of haloperidol and thioridazine in geriatric outpatients. J Clin Psychiatry 40:17–20, 1979

Salzman C: A primer on geriatric psychopharmacology. Am J Psychiatry 139:67–74, 1982

Salzman C: Treatment of agitation in the elderly, in Psychopharmacology: The Third Generation of Progress. Edited by Meltzer HY. New York, Raven, 1987, pp 1167–1176

Schneider LS, Pollock VE, Lyness SA: A metaanalysis of controlled trials of neuroleptic treatment in dementia. J Am Geriatr Soc 38:553–563, 1990

Schneider LS, Sobin PB: Non-neuroleptic medications in the management of agitation in Alzheimer's disease and other dementia: a selective review. International Journal of Geriatric Psychiatry 6:691–708, 1991

Seltzer B, Sherwin L: A comparison of early- and late-onset primary degenerative dementia. Arch Neurol 40:143–146, 1983

Shulman E, Steinberg G: Emotional reactions of Alzheimer's caregivers in support group settings (abstract). Gerontologist 24:158, 1984

Smith GR, Taylor CW, Linkous P: Haloperidol versus thioridazine for the treatment of psychogeriatric patients: a double-blind clinical trial. Psychosomatics 15:134–138, 1974

Steele C, Lucas M, Tune L: Haloperidol vs. thioridazine in the treatment of behavioral symptoms in senile dementia of the Alzheimer's type: preliminary findings. J Clin Psychiatry 47:310–312, 1986

Stotsky B: Multicenter studying thioridazine with diazepam and placebo in elderly, nonpsychotic patients with emotional and behavioral disorders. Clin Ther 6:546–559, 1984

Sugarman AA, Williams H, Alderstein AM: Haloperidol in the psychiatric disorders of old age. Am J Psychiatry 120:1190–1192, 1964

Sunderland T, Silver M: Neuroleptics in the treatment of dementia. International Journal of Geriatric Psychiatry 3:79–88, 1988

Tepper S, Haas J: Prevalence of tardive dyskinesia. J Clin Psychiatry 40:508–516, 1979

Terman L: Treatment of senile agitation with chlorpromazine. Geriatrics 10:520–522, 1955

Terry RD, Katzman R: Senile dementia of the Alzheimer type. Ann Neurol 14:497–506, 1983

Tewfik GI, Jain VK, Harcup M, et al: Effectiveness of various tranquilizers in the management of senile restlessness. Gerontology Clinics 12:351–359, 1970

Tobin JM, Brousseau ER, Lorenz AA: Clinical evaluation of haloperidol in geriatric patients. Geriatrics 25:119–122, 1970

Tsuang M, Lu LM, Stotsky BA, et al: Haloperidol versus thioridazine for hospitalized psychogeriatric patients: double-blind study. J Am Geriatr Soc 19:593–600, 1971

Tune LE, Steele C, Cooper T: Neuroleptic drugs in the management of behavioral symptoms of Alzheimer's disease. Psychiatr Clin North Am 14:353–73, 1991

Volavka J, Cooper TB: Review of haloperidol blood level and clinical response: looking through the window. J Clin Psychopharmacol 7:25–30, 1987

Wragg R, Jeste D: Neuroleptics and alternative treatments: management of behavioral symptoms and psychosis in Alzheimer's disease and related conditions. Psychiatr Clin North Am 11:195–212, 1988

Wragg RE, Jeste DV: Overview of depression and psychosis in Alzheimer's disease. Am J Psychiatry 146:577–587, 1989

CHAPTER 8

Use of Benzodiazepines in Behaviorally Disturbed Patients: Risk-Benefit Ratio

Shirish Patel, M.B.B.S., M.R.C.Psych.
Pierre N. Tariot, M.D.

*I*t is estimated that between 60% and 90% of patients with dementia of the Alzheimer type (DAT) have associated behavioral disturbances at some point in the course of the illness (Bozzola et al. 1992; Reisberg et al. 1989; Swearer et al. 1988; Tariot and Blazina 1994; Teri et al. 1989; Wragg and Jeste 1989). The etiologies of behaviors complicating DAT are unknown for the most part. The consequences of such behavioral disturbances, however, are legion and include psychological distress for the patient, the potential use (appropriate or inappropriate) of psychotropic medications, abuse of the patient and/or caregiver, institutionalization, and the use of restraints.

In this chapter we review the rational use of benzodiazepines in managing the symptoms of behaviorally disturbed DAT patients. The use of benzodiazepines in DAT must always be guided by a sound knowledge of the pharmacokinetics and pharma-

This work was supported in part by grants from the National Institute of Mental Health (K07MH00733 and P50MH40381).

codynamics of this class of drug and an understanding of the effect of age and disease on patients' sensitivity to the therapeutic and toxic effects of these agents.

Pharmacology of Benzodiazepines With Specific Reference to DAT

Benzodiazepines exert their effect by binding to specific benzodiazepine receptors located on the neuronal cell membranes in the brain (Mohler and Okada 1977). Age-related alterations in the benzodiazepine receptors (van der Kleijn et al. 1981) render older patients more sensitive to the effects of benzodiazepines, predisposing them to toxicity in doses that would cause no adverse effect in younger patients. Preexisting illnesses—for example, stroke and degenerative brain diseases such as DAT—also increase the risk of benzodiazepine drug toxicity.

Pharmacokinetics

Significant pharmacokinetic differences exist within the class of benzodiazepines. All the benzodiazepines are highly lipophilic and therefore cross the blood-brain barrier readily. The class of benzodiazepines can be broadly divided into the so-called long-acting and short-acting compounds. The long-acting compounds (e.g., diazepam, flurazepam) have a half-life longer than 24 hours and are catabolized to clinically active metabolites that require a hepatic cytochrome P-450 mixed-oxidase system for further degradation. The short-acting compounds (e.g., lorazepam, triazolam), on the other hand, generally have half-lives of less than 24 hours and have no active metabolites.

An awareness of these pharmacokinetic properties of benzodiazepines has clinical implications for prescribing for elderly DAT patients. For example, to obtain a rapid onset of action—as in the case of an agitated delirious patient—or to control seizures, diazepam, one of the most lipophilic benzodiazepines, is preferred over other drugs in its class. For situations demanding limited duration of action without any carryover effects—for example, insomnia—short-acting benzodiazepines are usually indicated. A short-acting benzodiazepine is also a logical choice in DAT patients who are taking other medications (e.g., cimetidine) that impair the hepatic cytochrome P-450 mixed-oxidase system. Because the short-acting benzodiazepines do not have active metabolites to be degraded by this enzyme system, the potential for toxicity resulting from active drug metabolites is virtually nil. On the other hand, for situations where prolonged administration of benzodiazepines is likely—for example, in a DAT patient with a preexisting and long-standing generalized anxiety state—long-acting benzodiazepines are more appropriate. Such a strategy allows for a once-a-day dose, and patients experience relatively fewer and less severe withdrawal symptoms on discontinuation of therapy with long-acting than with short-acting benzodiazepines (Salzman 1990).

The pharmacokinetics of benzodiazepines may be altered with increasing age of the patient. Benzodiazepines are largely bound to albumin in blood. Hypoalbuminemia is common in old age, with the result that a greater portion of the benzodiazepines remain unbound and therefore metabolically active. This result in turn predisposes to toxicity. With advancing age, there is also a slowing of hepatic metabolism. One consequence of this slowing is that the elimination half-life of the drugs metabolized by the liver is prolonged. With benzodiazepines, this consequence may cause toxicity from accumulation of the parent compound, particularly from long-acting benzodiazepines and their active metabolites. Finally, concomitant use of other medications, a very common occurrence in elderly people, may increase (e.g., cimetidine) or decrease (e.g., steroids) benzodiazepine blood levels, resulting in toxic or subtherapeutic effects, respectively.

Table 8–1 summarizes clinically relevant information regarding representative benzodiazepines.

Side Effects of Benzodiazepines in DAT

Benzodiazepines are generally well tolerated and have few side effects at therapeutic doses. In patients with DAT, however, the risks of adverse effects and toxicity are significantly increased as a result of the kinds of factors discussed above. The degenerative changes in the brains of patients with DAT leave these patients with a significantly reduced central compensatory reserve. Because DAT is primarily a disease of old age, the biological changes that accompany advancing age affect the pharmacokinetics and pharmacodynamics of benzodiazepines as discussed above, thereby enhancing the susceptibility of these patients to drug toxicity. Clinicians should also recognize that patients with DAT are quite often unable to convey their experiences of the side

Table 8–1.   Pharmacological profiles of some representative benzodiazepines

General name	Elimin- ation half-life	Usual dose (mg/day)	Comment
Short-acting			
Triazolam	2–6	0.125–0.250	Commonly prescribed hypnotic; significant risk of delirium
Temazepam	8–20	10–20	Useful hypnotic
Oxazepam	8–20	10–45	Low lypophilicity; useful sedative
Lorazepam	10–20	0.5–3.0	Useful in anxiety associated with physical illnesses; po, im, iv equally effective; anterograde amnesia common
Alprazolam	12–20	0.25–2.00	Debatable antidepressant properties; tolerance and withdrawal symptoms more commonly reported
Medazolam	1–12	1–4	Useful for acute sedation; available in parenteral forms only; significant anterograde amnesia common
Long-acting			
Diazepam	75–90	2–10	Useful sedative; advantage of qd or qod dosage
Chlordiaze- poxide	24–48	10–40	Ataxia common
Flurazepam	50–200	10–30	Risk of side effects high because of prolonged half-life

effects. This information should therefore be sought from their caregivers in terms of changes in the patients' behavior, and where possible, patients should be assessed for side effects.

Daytime sedation is the most common side effect reported with benzodiazepines. This adverse effect, more commonly associated with long-acting benzodiazepines, is usually dose-related. An *increased risk of falls* (Sorock and Shimken 1988) resulting in hip fractures has been associated with the use of long-acting benzodiazepines in elderly people (Ray et al. 1989). Chronic sedation with benzodiazepines also causes increased *confusion* and behavioral disturbances, including agitation, belligerence, and social disinhibition—symptoms that closely mimic behaviors complicating DAT. One needs to be aware of this because attempts to further sedate DAT patients in these situations by increasing the dose of benzodiazepines may lead to worse symptoms. In some patients, paradoxical rage reactions resulting from reduced inhibitions may be seen, particularly in those with a tendency toward aggressive behavior (Gaind and Jacoby 1978).

Almost all benzodiazepines, short-acting as well as long-acting, cause *anterograde amnesia* (Curran 1986; Lister 1985; Salzman 1990). In patients with baseline cognitive impairment such as DAT, this result causes further impairment of attention and short-term memory, leading in turn to increased confusion (Sunderland et al. 1989).

Withdrawal symptoms, including apprehension, tremor, and insomnia, are commonly reported after discontinuation of benzodiazepines, a result that precludes their prolonged use. The phenomena of rebound insomnia and rebound anxiety occur sooner and are more intense after withdrawal of short-acting benzodiazepines (Kales et al. 1986).

Other, less commonly reported side effects of benzodiazepines include signs of cerebellar toxicity like *ataxia, dysarthria,* and *incoordination* and signs of central nervous system depression, including *drowsiness, dizziness,* and *lightheadedness.*

Tolerance and Dependence

The issue of tolerance for and dependence on the sedative-hypnotic effects of benzodiazepines is controversial. An earlier report of tolerance for the hypnotic effect of triazolam (Kales et al. 1976) was not replicated in later studies (Leibowitz and Sunshine 1978; Mitler et al. 1984; Pegram et al. 1980). Subsequent studies also demonstrated sustained hypnotic efficacy of triazolam, flurazepam, and quazepam over several weeks (Kales et al. 1980, 1982; Mitler et al. 1984). On the other hand, development of tolerance to benzodiazepines is suggested by reports of gradual reduction in the intensity of daytime sedative effect with prolonged use of the drugs (Mitler et al. 1984) and by clinical impressions that these hypnotics lose their efficacy after 20–30 days of continuous use. The reluctance of elderly patients treated with low-dose benzodiazepine hypnotics to give up the drug (Kales and Kales 1984) and the continued use of the hypnotic in patients with chronic sleep disturbances, despite clinical evidence of lack of efficacy of the drug (Bixler et al. 1985), both support the notion that dependence on benzodiazepines does develop.

In summary, patients with DAT are at a greater risk of developing the side effects of benzodiazepines than are patients without this illness. The use of this class of psychotropic medication in these patients, therefore, should be determined in the context of the drug risk-benefit ratio.

Indications for the Use of Benzodiazepines in DAT

What are the possible indications for the use of benzodiazepines in DAT? It would be logical to consider using them in patients with a clear-cut anxiety syndrome, or at least some symptoms of anxiety—either free-floating or secondary to a time-limited stressor, such as admission to a hospital. Benzodiazepines also have a role in the management of insomnia. There is an occasional basis for their use in treating alcohol withdrawal syndromes in patients with dementia, in situations where time-limited sedation is desired—for example, before procedures, and for antipsychotic-induced akathisia in patients for whom ongoing antipsychotic therapy is necessary. Finally, benzodiazepines are sometimes used in a nonspecific fashion for agitation.

We now review the therapeutic role of benzodiazepines in the management of these behaviors complicating DAT.

Anxiety

The essential feature of anxiety is an excessive subjective sense of apprehension about real or perceived problems. Its prevalence in DAT has been reported to range between 0% and 50% (Baker et al. 1991; Patterson et al. 1990; Reisberg et al. 1989), with a median prevalence of about 32%. Anxiolytics are the mainstay of the pharmacotherapy of anxiety in other populations, and benzodiazepines are the most effective of the pharmacological interventions (Hershey and Kim 1988; Pinsker and Suljaga-Petchel 1984).

Systematic management of anxiety symptoms in DAT begins with the identification and correction of the underlying etiological factors. The list of factors precipitating or exacerbating anxiety is endless. Some of the more common causes, however, include physical illnesses, particularly cardiac dysrhythmias, chronic obstructive pulmonary disease, and hyperthyroidism; drugs, including caffeine, phenylpropanolamine (a common ingredient in over-the-counter cold remedies); psychiatric disorders, including depression and alcohol abuse or withdrawal; and environmental stressors. Particular attention should be paid to the presence of any depressive symptoms, because symptoms of anxiety are common in major depression. In such cases the appropriate therapy is antidepressant medication.

Agitation

In clinical practice, it is not uncommon for benzodiazepines to be used in patients experiencing nonspecific agitation. Using the "psychobehavioral metaphor" approach (Leibovici and Tariot 1988), it might be reasonable to consider using benzodiazepines, particularly in patients whose agitated symptoms can be interpreted as potentially anxiety-related, or at least overlapping with the anxiety symptoms—for example, extreme motor restlessness, trembling, autonomic symptoms, and expressed fearfulness or apprehension (which may be quite fragmented because of language deficits).

Once a decision is made to use benzodiazepine therapy for

nonspecific agitation, there is limited literature to guide the clinician. One study investigated the pharmacological treatment of behaviors complicating unspecified dementia (Coccaro et al. 1990). No studies targeted specific problems that could be expected to be responsive to benzodiazepines in particular (e.g., sleep, anxiety). There are, however, a number of other studies that have assessed the efficacy of various benzodiazepines, most commonly oxazepam, in the management of nonspecific behavioral disturbances complicating chronic brain syndrome (Beber 1965; DeLamos et al. 1965; Gerz 1964; Holiday and Mihlayi 1966), cerebral arteriosclerosis (Chesrow et al. 1965), senility (Covington 1975; Kirven and Montero 1973; Tewfik et al. 1970), neuropsychiatric disorders (Chesrow et al. 1962; Sanders 1965), nonpsychotic elderly patients (Stotsky 1984), and dementia (Fritz and Stewart 1990). One study assessed the efficacy of clonazepam in agitation complicating Alzheimer's disease (Ginsburg 1991).

Most of these studies suffer from significant methodological drawbacks, including the failure to use rigid diagnostic criteria, heterogeneity of the populations studied, the lack of operational definitions of the target symptoms, and the absence of comparable rating scales for the outcome measures. These factors make a meaningful comparison across the studies difficult and also prevent generalizing their findings to patients with DAT. With these qualifications in mind, the available studies are discussed below.

In an 8-week double-blind comparison trial of oxazepam, haloperidol, and diphenhydramine in 59 patients with dementia (37 with possible DAT) and clinically significant behavioral disturbances, oxazepam was found to be as efficacious as the other two medications in the control of agitated behavior and in the improvement of activities of daily living (ADL) (Coccaro et al. 1990). The improvement in behavioral control with oxazepam was modest, and the incidence of side effects was low. There are several merits to this study, including the use of acceptable scales to rate outcome measures; examining the effects of drugs on patients' ADL; and incorporating assessments from nursing staff, who most often know the patients best. The main drawback of this study is the lack of a placebo group, and the possible specificity of the effect in any diagnostic subgroup is not addressed.

Two very similar studies compared the efficacy of diazepam

and thioridazine in controlling behavioral problems in "geriatric patients with senility" (Covington 1975; Kirven and Montero 1973). In the study by Kirven and Montero, 56 patients were prescribed either diazepam or thioridazine for 4 weeks under double-blind conditions. The subjects' behaviors were rated on the Hamilton Anxiety Scale (Hamilton 1959) and the Nurses Observation Scale for Inpatient Evaluation (NOSIE) (Honigfeld et al. 1966). Global evaluations of the subjects' "overall severity of and change in mental illness" were also rated. Overall, the outcome was reported to be more positive with thioridazine, although diazepam was found equally effective in controlling the symptoms of insomnia, depressed mood, and agitation. The commonest side effect experienced by the diazepam group was drowsiness. The findings of the other study (Covington 1975) were very similar and also favored thioridazine over the benzodiazepine. It is interesting to note that none of the patients in the thioridazine group were reported to experience increased confusion, as might be expected given the pronounced anticholinergic side effects of this phenothiazine.

Several other studies also reported on the beneficial effects of oxazepam in controlling disturbed behavior in elderly patients with organic brain disease (Beber 1965; Chesrow et al. 1965; Gerz 1964; Sanders 1965; Tewfik et al. 1970). Oxazepam was shown to be the most effective in controlling symptoms of anxiety, tension, irritability, agitation, and insomnia; drowsiness was the most commonly reported side effect of oxazepam. There is also some evidence that oxazepam is most efficacious when administered for short periods of time, usually not exceeding 8 weeks (Sanders 1965).

In another study, the efficacy of oxazepam and chlordiazepoxide, a long-acting benzodiazepine, was compared in a double-blind, placebo-controlled, crossover study of 148 psychogeriatric patients (139 with cerebral arteriosclerosis) who showed behavioral problems (Chesrow et al. 1965). Oxazepam was found to reduce the behavioral symptoms by 70%–100% in 56% of the patients; only 23% of the chlordiazepoxide treatment group experienced a 70%–100% reduction in symptoms. The corresponding incidences of side effects were 55% in the oxazepam group and 41% in the chlordiazepoxide group. Drowsiness was the most common side effect reported with oxazepam use, and additional complaints of ataxia and edema were also reported with chlordiazepoxide use.

It appears from the literature that benzodiazepines may be most effective in patients who report subjective anxiety and have symptoms of high arousal, muscular tension, and autonomic hyperactivity. When such symptoms occur, pharmacological principles dictate time-limited use of benzodiazepines—for example, to help tide the patient over a crisis or to help the patient cope with anticipatory anxiety.

Case 1

Mrs. A, a 78-year-old married woman, was admitted from her home to a long-term care facility because her husband was no longer able to look after her. She had been experiencing increasing forgetfulness, disorientation, and difficulties with her ADL over the previous 6 years and carried a diagnosis of DAT. Soon after her admission to the facility, she became more confused and exhibited significant behavioral problems, including wandering into other residents' rooms, attempting to leave the floor, refusing to take her medications, and pacing up and down all day long.

To control her behavior, she was started on diazepam 2.5 mg po bid. Two weeks later she was reported as being still quite agitated, and her dose of diazepam was increased to 5 mg po bid. Her behavior was reported as more manageable in that she did not wander as much, but 1 week later she fell and broke her hip. She was quite heavily sedated with diazepam throughout her stay on the surgical floor. On return to the facility, she was seen by a psychiatrist, who promptly tapered her diazepam over a period of 1 week. A special nurse was assigned to her care, and her husband was encouraged to visit her as often as possible. She settled down fairly quickly. Her behavior mellowed to an acceptable level, her confusion diminished significantly, and she was able to participate in physical therapy and some group activities on the floor.

This case illustrates the risks of prescribing long-acting benzodiazepines too readily in DAT patients with behavioral problems. A more systematic approach to the management of this patient's behavioral problems would have been the awareness of the difficulties the patient was experiencing in adjusting to her totally strange environment. Nonpharmacological measures, together with judicious use of short-acting benzodiazepines for a brief period, could have facilitated the patient's transition from home to a health care facility. The case also illustrates the risks of increasing the dosage of benzodiazepines without evaluating the patient for the possible side effects of medications. Failure to do so can often lead to serious adverse consequences for the patient.

Sleep Disturbance

Disruption of sleep is another common complication of DAT in which benzodiazepines may have a specific therapeutic role (Mendels 1991; Walsh and Fillinham 1990). These disturbances may take the form of changes in the diurnal rhythm, the pattern, or the quality of sleep. The prevalence of sleep disturbances in patients with DAT is reported to be between 0% and 47% (Reisberg et al. 1989; Tariot and Blazina 1994; Teri et al. 1989), with a mean prevalence rate of 25%. Multiple nighttime awakenings is the most common sleep problem reported. Sleep disturbance in patients with DAT often leads to behavioral problems in the daytime, particularly agitation and aggressiveness.

Systematic management of sleep disturbance entails the identification and correction of underlying etiological factors. Some of the more common conditions contributing to insomnia include stress; pain; physical conditions like chronic obstructive pulmonary disease; use of stimulants like alcohol, coffee, over-the-counter nasal decongestants, and appetite suppressants; prescribed drugs, particularly antiarrhythmics and bronchodilators; and psychiatric disorders, including depression and anxiety. Nonpharmacological measures like physical exercise, relaxation techniques, and hot baths should be tried when appropriate. When a hypnotic is indicated, a benzodiazepine is usually the drug of choice, with chloral hydrate a useful alternative. Unfortunately, no studies examine the effects of benzodiazepines in sleep disturbances accompanying DAT. However, some general guidelines can be derived from studies of hypnotics in elderly people with sleep disturbance.

An ideal hypnotic would be one that shortens sleep latency (time to onset of sleep), eliminates nighttime awakenings, and is free from side effects, particularly daytime sedation. Although no such hypnotic exists, some of the short-acting benzodiazepines come closest to fulfilling these criteria. Triazolam, an ultra-short-acting benzodiazepine with a half-life of about 2–6 hours, causes rapid sleep induction by significantly shortening sleep latency, as determined by polysomnographic studies (Mendels 1991; Walsh and Fillinham 1990). This is perhaps the effect that has made triazolam the most frequently prescribed benzodiazepine hypnotic in the United States. However, an unusually high frequency of side effects has been reported with triazolam use in the general population (Bixler et al. 1987; Lasagna 1977), raising the possibility of even greater toxicity in patients with DAT. These side effects include delirium, anterograde amnesia, and automatic movements, collectively dubbed the "triazolam syndrome" (Patterson 1987). Serious concern about these side effects led to its withdrawal from the United Kingdom market (Dyer 1991). Another drawback of triazolam is rebound awakening occurring in the early hours of the morning as a result of the ultrashort half-life of the medication. This often necessitates repeating the dose at that time, which in turn may lead to daytime sedation, anxiety, irritability, and increased confusion.

A useful alternative hypnotic to triazolam is temazepam. Its efficacy is reported to be around 80% in patients of all ages; only about 7% of patients report carryover effects (Fowler 1980). Its side effect profile is similar to that of other short-acting benzodiazepines.

Theoretically, other short-acting benzodiazepines listed in Table 8–1 may also be prescribed as hypnotics, although there are not enough clinical data for these drugs to recommend their use. Medazolam, available only in parenteral form, should be reserved for patients who cannot take medicine orally and who require sedation (e.g., patients with delirium.)

Once a decision to prescribe a benzodiazepine hypnotic is made, particular attention should be paid to the known pharmacokinetics and pharmacodynamics of the drug chosen so that the needs of the individual patient are met. For instance, a patient who is experiencing significant difficulty in falling asleep requires a benzodiazepine that causes rapid sleep induction (e.g., triazolam), whereas for a patient who reports early morning waking, a benzodiazepine that covers the total duration of sleep is indicated (e.g., temazepam). Similarly, the dose of the prescribed drug should be individually tailored to achieve maximum clinical response and minimum or no side effects. The patient's response to the hypnotic should be assessed after the first night of prescription to decide whether the dose was adequate or excessive.

Benzodiazepine hypnotics should be prescribed for transient and short-term insomnia only (Committee on the Review of Medicines 1980; Consensus Conference 1984; White House Office of Drug Policy and National Institute on Drug Abuse 1979), because tolerance and cognitive impairment are known to develop with prolonged use. Tolerance to the benzodiazepine hypnotics, particularly the short-acting benzodiazepines (Salzman 1990), is a concern with continued use of the drug; the clinician should be alert to this, particularly in a patient who demands increasing doses of such a hypnotic. For this reason, some clinicians advocate intermittent use of the hypnotic (i.e., one to four times a week) (Gaillard 1987; Short-acting benzodiazepines 1987).

The role of long-acting benzodiazepines (e.g., flurazepam) in the management of insomnia should be restricted to patients in whom insomnia is associated with daytime agitation, where the carryover effects of the hypnotic could be beneficial. They may also be prescribed in selected patients in whom the withdrawal phenomena of rebound insomnia and rebound anxiety associated with short-acting benzodiazepines are unacceptable risks.

Case 2

Mr. S, a 76-year-old retired businessman, was brought to the outpatient clinic by his wife for evaluation and management of his sleep disturbance. Four years previously he had been diagnosed with DAT; at the time of his presentation he demonstrated significant impairments in both his short-term and his long-term memory, in his social judgment, and in his ability to care for himself. His wife reported that for the previous 4 weeks, her husband, who had been a reasonably good sleeper until then, had been waking up frequently at night to go to the bathroom. This would happen 6–10 times a night, and on returning to bed he would toss and turn and would rarely be able to sleep for any length of time. He would then nap during the day. He was often irritable and on several occasions had even threatened his wife with assault. She denied any recent change in her husband's routines or habits, in particular his use of alcohol or coffee.

Urinalysis revealed a urinary tract infection that cleared up with antibiotics. However, the patient continued to have frequent nighttime awakenings and was therefore prescribed temazepam 10 mg po q hs. The next day the patient's wife reported that he had slept "like a log," waking up only once during the night. Two days later she called again to say that although her husband was no longer waking up at night, he was slow, appeared drunk, and was frequently catnapping during the day. She was instructed to give him temazepam once every second or third night. Two weeks later, at the follow-up appointment, she said her husband was having "more good nights than bad nights" and that she gave him his pills on an average of twice a week.

This case illustrates the systematic management of sleep disturbance in a patient with DAT. Most likely, this patient's sleep disturbance was triggered by his urinary tract infection. The reason for the persistence of his nocturnal awakenings is not clear. The case also highlights the importance of tailoring the dose and the frequency of the hypnotic to an individual patient's needs.

Conclusions

The judicious and informed use of benzodiazepines can be helpful in the management of certain disturbed behaviors in DAT, notably insomnia, anxiety, and nonspecific agitation. Benzodiazepines should be used with caution, however, and for limited periods, always considering the risk-benefit ratio for the DAT patient. Pharmacological principles should guide the choice of agent and dosage, and the importance of careful observation of the target symptoms as well as of toxicity cannot be overemphasized. In view of the common association of symptoms of anxiety and depression in patients with DAT, a low threshold should exist for considering antidepressant therapy rather than the use of benzodiazepines. When treating either a specific or a nonspecific syndrome, it is of course always important to choose an appropriate time to perform the medication trial "in reverse," that is, gradually discontinuing the medication and observing the patient for withdrawal effects as well as for reemergence of the original target symptoms.

References

Baker F, Kokmen E, Chandra V, et al: Psychiatric symptoms in cases of clinically diagnosed Alzheimer's disease. J Geriatr Psychiatry Neurol 4:71–78, 1991

Beber C: Management of behavior in the institutionalized aged. Dis Nerv Syst 26:591–595, 1965

Bixler EO, Kales JD, Kales A, et al: Rebound insomnia and elimination half-life: assessment of individual subject response. J Clin Pharmacol 25:115–124, 1985

Bixler EO, Kales A, Brubaker BH, et al: Adverse reactions in benzodiazepine hypnotics: spontaneous reporting system. Pharmacology 35:286–300, 1987

Bozzola F, Gorelick P, Freels S: Personality changes in Alzheimer's disease. Arch Neurol 49:297–300, 1992

Chesrow EJ, Kaplitz SE, Breme JT, et al: Use of a new benzodiazepine derivative (Valium) in chronically ill and disturbed elderly patients. J Am Geriatr Soc 10:667–670, 1962

Chesrow EJ, Kaplitz SE, Vetra H, et al: Double-blind study of oxazepam in the management of geriatric patients with behavioral problems. Clin Med 72:1001–1005, 1965

Coccaro EF, Kramer E, Zemishlany Z, et al: Pharmacologic treatment of noncognitive behavioral disturbances in elderly demented patients. Am J Psychiatry 147:1640–1645, 1990

Committee on the Review of Medicines: Systematic review of the benzodiazepines: guidelines for data sheets on diazepam, chlordiazepoxide, medazepam, clorazepate, lorazepam, oxazepam, temazepam, triazolam, nitrazepam, and flurazepam. BMJ 280:910–912, 1980

Consensus Conference: Drugs and insomnia: the use of medications to promote sleep. Final report. JAMA 251:2410–2414, 1984

Covington JS: Alleviating agitation, apprehension, and related symptoms in geriatric patients: a double-blind comparison of phenothiazine and a benzodiazepine. South Med J 68:719–724, 1975

Curran HV: Tranquillising memories: a review of the effects of benzodiazepines on human memory. Biol Psychol 23:179–213, 1986

DeLamos GP, Clements WR, Nickels E: Effect of diazepam suspension in geriatric patients hospitalized for psychiatric illness. J Am Geriatr Soc 13:355–359, 1965

Dyer C: Halcion banned in U.K. BMJ 303:877, 1991

Fowler LK: Post-marketing surveillance of Euhypnos (temazepam). J Int Med Res 8:295–299, 1980

Fritz J, Stewart JT: Lorazepam treatment of resistive aggression in dementia (letter). Am J Psychiatry 147:1250, 1990

Gaillard JM: Place of benzodiazepines in the treatment of sleep disturbances. Rev Med Suisse Romande 107:717–720, 1987

Gaind R, Jacoby R: Benzodiazepines causing aggression, in Current Themes in Psychiatry I. Edited by Gaind RN, Hudson BL. London, Macmillan, 1978, pp 371–379

Gerz HO: A preliminary report on the management of geriatric patients with oxazepam. Am J Psychiatry 120:1110–1111, 1964

Ginsburg ML: Clonazepam for agitated patients with Alzheimer's disease. Can J Psychiatry 36:237–238, 1991

Hamilton M: The assessment of anxiety states by rating. Br J Med Psychol 32:50–55, 1959

Hershey LA, Kim KY: Diagnosis and treatment of anxiety in the elderly. Rational Drug Therapy 22:1–6, 1988

Holiday AR, Mihlayi E: A controlled evaluation of two dose levels of oxazepam compared to placebo. Journal of New Drugs 6:124–132, 1966

Honigfeld G, Gillis RC, Klett CJ: NOSIE-30: a treatment-sensitive ward behavior scale. Psychol Rep 19:180–182, 1966

Kales A, Kales JD: Evaluation and Treatment of Insomnia. New York, Oxford University Press, 1984, pp 263–265

Kales A, Kales J, Bixler EO, et al: Hypnotic efficacy of triazolam: sleep laboratory evaluation of intermediate-term effectiveness. J Clin Pharmacol 16:399–406, 1976

Kales A, Scharf MB, Soldatos CR, et al: Quazepam, a new benzodiazepine hypnotic: intermediate sleep laboratory evaluation. J Clin Pharmacol 20:184–192,1980

Kales A, Bixler EO, Soldatos CR, et al: Quazepam and fluorazepam: long-term use and extended withdrawal. Clin Pharmacol Ther 32:781–788, 1982

Kales A, Bixler EO, Vela-Bueno A, et al: Comparison of short and long half-life benzodiazepine hypnotics: triazolam and quazepam. Clin Pharmacol Ther 40:378–386, 1986

Kirven LE, Montero EF: Comparison of thioridazine and diazepam in the control of nonpsychotic symptoms associated with senility: double-blind study. J Am Geriatr Soc 21:546–551, 1973

Lasagna L: The role of benzodiazepines in non-psychiatric medical practice. Am J Psychiatry 134:656–658, 1977

Leibovici A, Tariot PN: Agitation associated with dementia: a systematic approach to treatment. Psychopharmacol Bull 24:49–53, 1988

Leibowitz M, Sunshine A: Long-term hypnotic efficacy and safety of triazolam (Halcion) and flurazepam (Dalmane). J Clin Pharmacol 18:302–309, 1978

Lister RG: The amnesic action of benzodiazepines in man. Neurosci Biobehav Rev 9:87–94, 1985

Mendels J: Criteria for selection of appropriate benzodiazepine hypnotic therapy. J Clin Psychiatry 52 (suppl 9):42–46, 1991

Mitler MM, Seidel WF, van den Hoed J, et al: Comparative hypnotic effects of flurazepam, triazolam and placebo: a long-term simultaneous nighttime and daytime study. J Clin Psychopharmacol 4:2–16, 1984

Mohler H, Okada T: Benzodiazepine receptor: demonstration in the central nervous system. Science 198:849–851, 1977

Patterson JF: Triazolam syndrome in the elderly. South Med J 80:1425–1426, 1987

Patterson M, Schnell A, Martin R, et al: Assessment of behavioral and affective symptoms in Alzheimer's disease. J Geriatr Psychiatry Neurol 3:21–30, 1990

Pegram V, Hyde P, Linton P: Chronic use of triazolam: the effects on the sleep patterns of insomniacs. J Int Med Res 8:224–231, 1980

Pinsker H, Suljaga-Petchel K: Use of benzodiazepines in primary-care geriatric patients. J Am Geriatr Soc 32:595–598, 1984

Ray WA, Griffin MR, Downey W: Benzodiazepines of long and short elimination half-life and the risk of hip fracture. JAMA 262:3303–3307, 1989

Reisberg B, Franssen E, Sclan S, et al: State specific incidence of potentially remediable behavioral symptoms in aging and Alzheimer's disease: a study of 120 patients using the BEHAVE-AD. Bull Clin Neurosci 54:95–112, 1989

Salzman C: Benzodiazepine toxicity, in Benzodiazepine Dependence, Toxicity, and Abuse: A Task Force Report of the American Psychiatric Association. Washington, DC, American Psychiatric Association, 1990, pp 41–48

Sanders JF: Evaluation of oxazepam and placebo in emotionally disturbed aged patients. Geriatrics 20:739–749, 1965

Short-acting benzodiazepines: to prescribe or not to prescribe? (editorial) Union Med Can 29:116, 1987

Sorock GS, Shimken EE: Benzodiazepine sedative and the risk of falling in a community-dwelling elderly cohort. Arch Intern Med 148:2441–2444, 1988

Stotsky B: Multicenter study comparing thioridazine with diazepam and placebo in elderly, nonpsychotic patients with emotional and behavioral disorders. Clin Ther 6:546–559, 1984

Sunderland T, Weingartner H, Cohen R, et al: Low-dose oral lorazepam administration in Alzheimer subjects and age-matched controls. Psychopharmacology 99:129–133, 1989

Swearer JM, Drachman DA, O'Donnell BF, et al: Troublesome and disruptive behaviors in dementia. J Am Geriatr Soc 36:784–790, 1988

Tariot P, Blazina L: The psychopathology of dementia, in Handbook of Dementing Illnesses. Edited by Morris J. New York, Marcel Dekker, 1994, pp 461–476

Teri L, Borsen S, Kiyak H, et al: Behavioral disturbance, cognitive dysfunction, and functional skills. Prevalence in relationship to Alzheimer's disease. J Am Geriatr Soc 37:109–116, 1989

Tewfik GI, Jain VK, Harcup M, et al: Effectiveness of various tranquilizers in the management of senile restlessness. Gerontol Clin 12:351–359, 1970

van der Kleijn E, Vree TB, Baars AM, et al: Factors influencing the activity and fate of benzodiazepines in the elderly. Br J Clin Pharmacol 11:85S–98S, 1981

Walsh JK, Fillinham JM: Role of hypnotic drugs in general practice. Am J Med 99:34–38, 1990

White House Office of Drug Policy and National Institute on Drug Abuse: FDA Drug Bulletin, August 1979, p 16

Wragg R, Jeste D: Overview of depression and psychosis in Alzheimer's disease. Am J Psychiatry 146:577–587, 1989

CHAPTER 9

Treatment of Depression

Michael Serby, M.D.

*D*epression, a frequent complication of Alzheimer's disease, may be a potentially remediable and reversible component of an otherwise untreatable illness. When considering whether to treat depression complicating dementia, the risk-benefit ratio of intervention in each individual case must be examined. Although the successful treatment of depression might be expected to improve functional ability and quality of life in Alzheimer's disease patients, little empirical evidence supports this view. However, it is extremely difficult to quantify the improvement in well-being or quality of life that might accrue from successful treatment of depression in Alzheimer's disease patients, and the lack of efficacy data should not necessarily deter active treatment of these patients.

On the other hand, there are a number of compelling reasons to be clinically conservative in the use of antidepressants in Alzheimer's disease. In depressed patients who are otherwise healthy, a trial of a drug can often be justified because there is limited risk. However, patients with dementia frequently develop increased memory impairment while on antidepressants. In fact, in the only controlled trial to date on this subject, antidepressant treatment produced greater cognitive decline than did placebo (Reifler et al. 1989). For this reason, a cautious approach to pharmacological intervention for this patient population should be adopted.

In this chapter I review the literature on the treatment of depression in the case of dementia, and I present a balanced management approach based on a critical assessment of the risk-benefit ratio.

General Considerations

Before treatment is begun, the patient must be thoroughly assessed. The diagnosis of depression must be reviewed, and the presence of delirium or medical comorbidity should be excluded as a possible cause of the affective disturbance. Furthermore, a careful and thorough review must be made of medications that could be contributing to the clinical picture. Both medical and social factors, in addition to the degree of depression, will determine whether hospitalization, a day hospital, or outpatient management is indicated. Although increasing confusion may be a possible reason to admit a patient, it must be balanced against the risk that the novel environment of a ward could exacerbate confusion. Once the venue for treatment is decided, a specific therapeutic modality, or a combination of strategies, can be determined.

Specific Approaches

Antidepressants

Although there is widespread anecdotal evidence for the successful treatment of depression in Alzheimer's disease with antidepressants, scientifically controlled studies in this area are virtually nonexistent. A retrospective chart review of antidepressant use in Alzheimer's disease patients suggested that approximately 85% of Alzheimer's disease patients with major depression responded favorably to treatment (Reifler et al. 1986). However, a double-blind comparison of imipramine (mean dose 83 mg/day) versus placebo found that drug and placebo treatments resulted in an equally significant decrease in depression scores (Reifler et al. 1989). Furthermore, active drug treatment resulted in greater cognitive decline than did the placebo. Thus, despite anecdotal evidence, few empirical data support the use of antidepressants in depressed Alzheimer's disease patients. Likewise, there are no controlled data on the most appropriate choice of antidepressant in this population, and currently this choice can only be guided by clinical judgment and clinician preference.

However, a number of points should be taken into consideration when choosing an antidepressant for an Alzheimer's disease patient. First, an agent with low anticholinergic potential is preferable. Alzheimer's disease patients are twice as sensitive to the cognition-impairing effects of anticholinergic agents (Sunderland et al. 1987) and are therefore at risk of developing delirium when taking highly anticholinergic tricyclics. In general, low doses of secondary amine derivatives, such as desipramine and nortriptyline, are preferred to the more anticholinergic tertiary amines, such as amitriptyline and imipramine.

Another potential catastrophic effect of tricyclic use in frail elderly dementia patients is the development of postural hypotension. Nortriptyline is less likely to have this adverse effect, and it is therefore the tricyclic of first choice in this population. Careful monitoring of postural blood pressure changes is of course warranted when tricyclics are prescribed to elderly patients with dementia.

Several reports have supported the use of monoamine oxidase inhibitors (MAOIs) in the treatment of depression complicating dementia (Ashford and Ford 1979; Jenike 1985, 1986). The fact that brain monoamine oxidase (MAO) levels increase with age and in particular with dementia (Adolfsson et al. 1980) provides some rationale for the utility of these agents in Alzheimer's disease patients. There has been particular interest in selegiline, a selective MAO-B inhibitor, because of its reported behavioral effects in Alzheimer's disease (Tariot et al. 1987). However, there is no evidence for antidepressant activity at the low doses of selegiline (5–10 mg) used in Alzheimer's disease. At these doses, the drug is a selective MAO-B inhibitor, whereas at higher antidepressant doses (30–60 mg) selegiline becomes a mixed MAO-A and MAO-B inhibitor, creating the same potential for side effects as with the more classic MAOIs. These include postural hypotension, insomnia, and the uncommon but dangerous hypertensive crisis, or "cheese reaction." Concern about these crises requires special dietary and medication restrictions that may be difficult to enforce in the forgetful patient, making the use of MAOIs somewhat riskier. The case reports suggesting the antidepressant efficacy of MAOIs in Alzheimer's disease patients will need to be confirmed in large controlled studies.

Psychostimulants were also reported to have a role in the treatment of depressed Alzheimer's disease patients (Woods et al. 1986), producing marked improvement in three of six patients with major depression and dementia but only moderate improvement in two of eight with dementia with depressive features. This distinction may be fruitful in future treatment studies. It should be noted that two patients with dementia became more confused during a stimulant trial but that the dementia was completely reversed when the drug was withdrawn. There were no cardiac side effects in this study, suggesting a favorable risk-benefit ratio if efficacy is confirmed. Although the limited studies do not warrant a recommendation of these agents without further research, low-dose stimulants may be considered as a treatment option in resistant cases.

Trazodone, a heterocyclic antidepressant, and the newer selective serotonin reuptake inhibitors (SSRIs) such as fluoxetine and sertraline have a favorable side effect profile for elderly dementia patients. The SSRIs in particular are free of anticholinergic side effects and have no clinically significant adverse effects on blood pressure or cardiac conduction. The agitation, restlessness, and gastrointestinal complaints produced by the SSRIs are generally not problematic at the low doses prescribed in Alzheimer's disease, but they may necessitate a different drug in some patients. Interestingly, SSRIs may exacerbate parkinsonian symptoms, a real consideration in some Alzheimer's disease patients because of reduced striatal dopamine levels (Winblad et al. 1982).

Bupropion, another novel antidepressant devoid of anticholinergic side effects, may be a useful adjunct to the pharmacological armamentarium in the treatment of depression complicating dementia. This agent may produce seizures in patients with organic brain disease, but the effect usually occurs at higher doses than are recommended in Alzheimer's disease. Excessive stimulation, including insomnia, is another potential pitfall with this drug.

Alterations in pharmacokinetics and particularly pharmacodynamics in elderly patients take on special significance in Alzheimer's disease, calling for conservative dosing strategies. It is best to start with very low doses and proceed cautiously. The agents used to treat depression in Alzheimer's disease and their dosage ranges are shown in Table 9–1.

For Alzheimer's disease patients with comorbid depression, there are no data to suggest appropriate strategies in patients who fail to respond to an antidepressant drug. The use of drug combinations or augmentation with thyroid or lithium must be viewed with caution until appropriate controlled studies can be conducted.

Table 9–1. Drugs used to treat depression complicating dementia

Drug class	Dose (mg)	Common side effects
Tricyclics		
Desipramine	50–150	Dry mouth, constipation, urinary
Nortriptyline	10–75	hesitancy, postural hypotension, conduction block
MAOIs		
Phenelzine	15–45	Postural hypotension, "cheese
Tranylcypromine	10–30	reaction"
Heterocyclics		
Trazodone	50–200	Hypotension, sedation
SSRIs		
Fluoxetine	10–20	Nausea, agitation, insomnia
Sertraline	50–100	Nausea
Paroxetine	10–30	Nausea
Atypicals		
Bupropion	100–200	Seizures, insomnia

Case 1

Mr. A, an 85-year-old man, was brought for treatment by his wife because of memory impairment for 1 year and possible depressive symptoms over a period of 6–8 months. His gradual onset and linear course of cognitive slippage and his workup were consistent with a diagnosis of probable Alzheimer's disease by the criteria of the National Institute of Neurological and Communicative Disorders and Stroke (NINCDS) (McKhann et al. 1984). He had withdrawn from all activities and expressed no desire to live. His sleep was increased, but his appetite was poor, with a resultant 10-pound weight loss. Mr. A reported "no desire to do anything" and admitted feeling "very, very depressed." His Mini-Mental State Exam (MMSE) score was 18. A trial of nortriptyline began at a dose of 10 mg/day and was increased to 20 mg in a few days. At first his wife noted affective improvement, but the dose had to be reduced to 10 mg as a result of "dizziness" and then discontinued after 1 month because of vivid visual hallucinations and worsening confusion. These symptoms cleared once the nortriptyline was discontinued.

This case illustrates some potential problems of tricyclic use in this population. The most important side effect noted in this patient, the emergence of delirium, was undoubtedly related to the cholinergic blockade produced. The importance of slow, careful management, with low doses, is underscored.

Case 2

Ms. B, a 65-year-old woman, was brought by her daughter for evaluation of a combined cognitive and mood disorder of 1 year's duration. The patient had cared for her husband for 4 years as he deteriorated with Alzheimer's disease until he was placed in a nursing home. After his placement, Ms. B developed word-finding difficulties and became very forgetful. She also had significant vegetative changes and ruminative guilty thoughts. Her MMSE score was 17. A workup of her dementia was consistent with probable Alzheimer's disease. Fluoxetine (20 mg daily) resulted in a complete response of her melancholic symptoms within 1 month; this response has been sustained through several months of treatment. The patient's cognitive deficits were unaffected, however, and her MMSE score remains 15 despite her euthymic state.

The use of SSRIs in this case resulted in a therapeutic outcome free of side effects. Despite the reported emergence of symptoms after a traumatic life change, the patient did not seem to have a "pseudodementia" related to the depression. It may be that her children failed to notice her early symptoms because they were confronted with the more extreme disturbances in their father. The fact that her cognition did not improve after successful antidepressant treatment is consistent with a true dementia. This is the usual outcome in a mixed dementia-depression case; the effectiveness of treatment for depression does not generally extend to cognition.

Electroconvulsive Therapy

Electroconvulsive therapy (ECT) has also been used to treat depression in Alzheimer's disease. A number of case reports extol the virtues of this approach (DeMuth and Rand 1980; Price and McAllister 1989; Snow and Wells 1981), and one retrospective study comparing ECT in depressed Alzheimer's disease patients to ECT in elderly depressed people without dementia (Nelson and Rosenberg 1991) also supports the clinical benefit of ECT in depressed Alzheimer's disease patients. The evidence in this latter study suggested that patients with dementia may develop more confusion following ECT, but that this is a brief clinical issue. Interestingly, 21 Alzheimer's disease patients responded as well to a course of ECT as did 84 elderly depressed people (Nelson and Rosenberg 1991). No study has adequately addressed the relative risk-benefit ratio of unilateral versus bilateral ECT in this population. The general approach has been to start with unilateral treatments and to change to bilateral ECT if necessary. However, the unilateral approach probably requires more treatments, raising the specter of greater risk due to anesthesia and cardiac consequences in this elderly population.

A word of caution is warranted, given the aggressive use of ECT in some quarters. It is important not to misconstrue withdrawal and agitation in a dementia patient, in the absence of true affective changes, as melancholia. The use of ECT in such circumstances is unwarranted, and it is likely to make the patient more confused and agitated.

Case 3

Mrs. C, an 87-year-old woman, was transferred from her nursing home residence to a private hospital because of increased agitation. Neuroleptic management resulted in a decrease in activity to a point described as depression by the attending psychiatrist, who recommended ECT. A second opinion was sought by the family. The patient was very confused and apathetic, but she showed no sign of sadness or tearfulness. Her MMSE score was 0. This clinical picture weighed against the use of ECT.

Psychotherapy for Depression in the Face of Dementia

In the imipramine double-blind study, placebo treatment was equivalent to the administration of imipramine in terms of antidepressant efficacy, with a clear-cut improvement in both conditions (Reifler et al. 1989). One may conclude that the clinic visits themselves were therapeutic, but the specific type of intervention is unclear. There is no question that psychotherapy in a general sense is an important tool in Alzheimer's disease complicated by depression and that regular visits to the clinic or office may be beneficial in many ways. It is possible, for example, that this serves as an activity for the patient, who feels positive about the experience with family and other obviously concerned people. The therapist may directly communicate to the patient in clear, supportive terms, a repetitive process that can be successful to a degree. Cognitive and behavioral techniques are advocated by some geriatricians (Teri and Gallagher-Thompson 1991). Specific approaches include the identification of pleasant activities, which are then increased (Teri and Logsdon 1991).

Family involvement in the therapeutic process is of paramount importance. Dysphoria and helplessness in caregivers exacerbate depression in the patient. It is important to provide tangible management guidelines, such as the need for structure, ease, and simplicity in the patient's routine (Weiner et al. 1991). Family members also need help in identifying those of their own issues that may have an impact on the patient. Unresolved conflicts may be heated up unilaterally, with the relative viewing the patient as recalcitrant or passive-aggressive or seeing him or her in some other equally hostile fashion. An educative approach, distinguishing between baseline character and behavior that is part of the dementia, should be launched. It is also important to address family ambivalence about placement decisions. It is likely that the major effect of therapy in Alzheimer's disease complicated by depression is achieved via these family-targeted interventions.

Conclusions

The treatment of depression in Alzheimer's disease requires a specialized approach by the psychiatrist. Diagnostic dilemmas must be resolved before treatment can begin. The use of medications and ECT may be helpful, but there are few data available by which to judge their efficacy with certainty. In any event, biological interventions must be used judiciously, with careful attention to side effects. Productive psychotherapy consists of supportive and cognitive-behavior techniques with the patient. Family interventions are often most critical, and the therapist should be easily available to caregivers, frequently by telephone, for the duration of their clinical needs.

An effective antidepressant response in Alzheimer's disease represents a rare positive step in a disease process otherwise characterized by an inexorable downward course. Given this clinical scenario, and the dearth of information on this topic, it is imperative that further studies be conducted to test and develop effective treatments for depression complicating Alzheimer's disease.

References

Adolfsson R, Gottfries CG, Oreland L, et al: Increased activity of brain and platelet monoamine oxidase in dementia of Alzheimer type. Life Sci 27:1029–1034, 1980

Ashford JW, Ford CV: Use of MAO inhibitors in elderly patients. Am J Psychiatry 136:1466–1467, 1979

DeMuth GW, Rand BS: Atypical major depression in a patient with severe primary degenerative dementia. Am J Psychiatry 137:1609–1610, 1980

Jenike MA: Monoamine oxidase inhibitors as treatment for depressed patients with primary degenerative dementia (Alzheimer's disease). Am J Psychiatry 142:763–764, 1985

Jenike MA: Use of MAOIs for demented depressed patients (letter). Am J Psychiatry 143:254, 1986

McKhann G, Drachman D, Folstein M, et al: Clinical diagnosis of Alzheimer's disease: report of the NINCDS-ADRDA Work Group under the auspices of Department of Health and Human Services Task Force on Alzheimer's Disease. Neurology 34:939–944, 1984

Nelson JP, Rosenberg DR: ECT treatment of demented elderly patients with major depression: a retrospective study of efficacy and safety. Convulsive Therapy 7:157–165, 1991

Price TPR, McAllister TW: Safety and efficacy of ECT in depressed patients with dementia: a review of clinical experience. Convulsive Therapy 5:61–74, 1989

Reifler BV, Larson E, Teri L, et al: Dementia of the Alzheimer's type and depression. J Am Geriatr Soc 34:855–859, 1986

Reifler BV, Teri L, Raskind M, et al: A double blind trial of a tricyclic antidepressant in Alzheimer's patients with and without depression. Am J Psychiatry 146:45–49, 1989

Snow SS, Wells CE: Case studies in neuropsychiatry: diagnosis and treatment of coexistent dementia and depression. J Clin Psychiatry 42:439–441, 1981

Sunderland T, Tariot PN, Cohen RM, et al: Anticholinergic sensitivity in patients with dementia of the Alzheimer type: a dose response study. Arch Gen Psychiatry 44:418–426, 1987

Tariot PN, Cohen RM, Sunderland T, et al: L-Deprenyl in Alzheimer's disease. Arch Gen Psychiatry 44:427–433, 1987

Teri L, Gallagher-Thompson D: Cognitive-behavioral interventions for treatment of depression in Alzheimer's patients. Gerontologist 31:413–416, 1991

Teri L, Logsdon RG: Identifying pleasant activities for Alzheimer's disease patients: the Pleasant Event Schedule—AD. Gerontologist 31:124–127, 1991

Weiner MF, Bruhn M, Svetlik D, et al: Experiences with depression in a dementia clinic. J Clin Psychiatry 52:234–238, 1991

Winblad B, Adolfsson R, Carlsson A, et al: Biogenic amines in brain of patients with Alzheimer's disease, in Alzheimer's Disease: A Report of Progress in Research. Edited by Corkin S, Davis KL, Growdon JH, et al. New York, Raven, 1982, pp 25–33

Woods SW, Tesar GE, Murray GB, et al: Psychostimulant treatment of depressive disorders secondary to initial illness. J Clin Psychiatry 47:12–15, 1986

CHAPTER 10

Nonpharmacological Treatment of Behavioral Symptoms

Gregory R. J. Swanwick, M.B., M.R.C.P.I., M.R.C.Psych.

*T*he majority of patients with dementia of the Alzheimer type (DAT) are cared for in the community by family or friends (Alessi 1991). Disruptive behaviors are therefore of critical importance, often resulting in reduced quality of life for the patient, increased burdens on the caregiver, and detrimental effects on personal relationships. Failure to cope with behavioral symptoms often precipitates institutionalization (Roper et al. 1991; Teri et al. 1988), with further effects on the needs of the agitated person and the other residents within the institution and with the possibility of overuse of physical and chemical restraints (Roper et al. 1991). A review of nursing home surveys reported a mean prevalence of disruptive behavior of 42.8% (Beck et al. 1991). Pillemer and Moore (1989) reported that between 70% and 80% of staff had been assaulted by nursing home residents. Overall, the available data suggest that approximately 70%–80% of patients with DAT manifest disruptive behavior in some form (Wragg and Jeste 1988). However, despite the fact that these behaviors often pose more critical management problems than memory or cognitive impairments in DAT, it is the latter that have been the main focus of dementia research.

The Need to Develop Nonpharmacological Strategies

A detailed literature review of agitated behaviors in dementia patients revealed that most studies are of a pharmacological or descriptive type (Cohen-Mansfield and Billig 1986) and that very few are systematic studies of behavioral or environmental interventions (Deutsch and Rovner 1991). Despite this, the efficacy of neuroleptics, the most widely used drugs for behavioral symptoms, is far from unequivocal (Wragg and Jeste 1988). Neuroleptics also have the risk of significant side effects. They include anticholinergic effects, cardiovascular toxicity, and extrapyramidal syndromes, some of which (e.g., akathisia) may be mistaken for agitation and may result in further medication (Thomas 1988). In the United States, recognition of these difficulties has resulted in federal legislation restricting the use of neuroleptics and restraints in nursing homes—the Omnibus Budget Reconciliation Act of 1987—which came into effect in 1990 (Rovner et al. 1992). Prescribing a neuroleptic now requires specific diagnoses and behavioral indications.

Clearly, pharmacological approaches can have significant human and economic costs, and nonpharmacological interventions should be considered the foundation of management for behavioral symptoms in DAT (Eimer 1989). Particular emphasis should be placed on the education and support of families, environmental and behavioral interventions, the formation of Alzheimer units in nursing homes, and the use of psychotropic agents only as an adjunct and to treat well-defined target symptoms (Deutsch and Rovner 1991; Eimer 1989). Chandler (1987) has proposed four basic principles of behavioral management: work with the family, environmental control, maintenance of routine, and environmental safety. I discuss these and other aspects of nonpharmacological management, along with suggested interventions for specific behavioral symptoms.

Nonpharmacological Management Strategies

Work With the Family

Understanding the emotional reaction of families and caregivers to the diagnosis and behavioral symptoms of DAT is essential to successful management, and the interpretation of some behaviors in DAT can be as critical as the disturbance itself (Roper et al. 1991). Particularly when premorbid relationships have been poor, the caregiver may interpret behaviors such as repetitive questioning as being deliberately annoying. Misinterpretations are also more likely to occur as the patient's verbal communication skills deteriorate. For example, a patient may take off his clothes or grab at a caregiver in an effort to express a need to go to the bathroom or because of pain. The caregiver could easily misinterpret these behaviors as either aggressive or of a sexual nature. Family therapy may be indicated to help families resolve feelings and adjust to changing roles (Jeste and Krull 1991), and it may also be of direct benefit in the management of behavioral symptoms. It is well known that the family or caregiver can significantly affect the patient's behavior. For example, patients with DAT are very sensitive to body language and to the tone of voice, especially when it conveys a criticism—even when they are no longer able to understand the specific content of the message (Knopman and Sawyer-DeMaris 1990).

Behavioral disturbance may also be the result of living with a dysfunctional family. Although family interventions can help the situation, and there is a desire on the part of helath care professsionals and informal caregivers to keep patients with their families, removal of a patient from such a stressful environment may be necessary (Eimer 1989). In addition, caregivers, including those in institutions, must carefully examine their own reactions to behavioral symptoms, because these responses may lead to actions that can increase the frequency or intensity of the problem (Roper et al. 1991). For example, as the ability to carry out activities of daily living deteriorates, patients need help with washing and other basic functions that were previously done in private. This may cause embarrassment for patients (and for caregivers) and result in agitation or resistance. The embarrassment should be recognized and efforts made to avoid it. (Some patients are less embarrassed when a stranger such as a "home help" helps with bathing, whereas others respond best to the primary caregiver.) If such efforts are not made, caregivers may resort unnecessarily to restraint and actually worsen the behavior.

Family interventions may best be approached by a multidisciplinary team; it must be recognized, however, that as the dementia progresses, family issues will change (Warshaw 1990). Education soon after diagnosis encourages family involvement and helps caregivers provide more accurate collateral information (Winograd and Jarvik 1986). Initial issues include failure to accept the diagnosis or prognosis, with the consequent risk of pushing patients to try harder and exacerbating the behavioral disturbance. At this stage, family meetings can be held to assess previous interpersonal relationships, responsibilities for care, and current community and family supports. This step should be followed by education and discussion regarding coping strategies, role changes, environmental manipulations, informal and formal supports, legal and financial considerations, and whatever other issues the families bring up. It is also useful to provide a reading list with a number of publications containing practical information aimed at families (e.g., Gidley and Shears 1988; Mace and Rabins 1981; Murphy 1986; New York City Alzheimer's Resource Center 1985; Powell and Courtice 1983; Reisberg 1983; Watt and Calder 1981; Wilcock 1990; Woods 1989).

In the middle stages, issues that need to be addressed are the grieving process, ethical issues involving conflict between safety and allowing autonomy, and increases in behavioral disturbances and caregiver burdens. Bereavement counseling and increased supports (e.g., family support groups such as those organized by the Alzheimer's Association, day care programs, and respite care) may be appropriate where available. In the final stages, terminal care and guilt at "abandonment" to institutionalization are likely issues. The family can be helped to locate and assess long-term care facilities and to discuss further role changes, feelings of guilt or relief at institutionalization, and how to deal most appropriately with visiting their relative.

Families vary in their capacity to cope with behavioral symptoms. At one end of the spectrum, some appear to adjust well and reach solutions on their own. At the other end are those who need considerable guidance. For the latter group, referral to a therapist trained in behavioral management techniques may be appropriate (Teri and Logsdon 1990). Teaching caregivers to identify behaviors, their antecedent stressors, and consequent events can prevent problem behaviors and catastrophic reactions (Alessi 1991).

Holidays and family occasions can often result in worsened behavioral disturbance for patients with DAT, but if their behavior is understood in terms of an inability to adapt to unfamiliar situations, efforts can be made to prevent or limit possible problems (Warshaw 1990). Some principles and suggestions, illustrated with clinical vignettes, are discussed here.

> John, a 72-year-old man with DAT, and his wife, Sheila, are to celebrate their 50th wedding anniversary. Their daughter wants to mark the occasion with dinner at an expensive restaurant with all their friends and large family. Sensibly, Sheila suggests that they have two smaller celebrations at home. Their relatives will be invited to one and close friends who are aware of John's limitations to the other. In this way John will be in a situation that he is familiar with and will not be confronted with a sea of faces that he is expected to recognize. In addition, Sheila and John will be able to go over old photographs and mementos that relate to the guests before they arrive, and this may help to orient John and avoid confusion.

Families often ask whether they should go along with mistakes or confused thinking or whether they should correct the person. In general, neither approach is advisable. Instead, the key to managing such situations is to reinforce any information that is accurate, very gently correct any that is wrong, and distract the person to something else if necessary.

> On Friday, Peter (a 60-year-old man with mild DAT) says to his son, "It's one o'clock. Time to go to the football game." Rather than directly correcting him, his son responds, "Yes, it is one o'clock" (agreeing with the accurate part), "but it's Friday and the game is on Saturday" (gentle correction), "so let's go shopping instead" (diversion).

> Mary, who has been in an Alzheimer unit for a 3-week period of respite care, is due to go home today. She repeatedly insists to the staff that she must go and collect her daughter from boarding school for the holidays. Mary knows that she is to see her daughter again today and that there is to be some sort of change in living arrangements.

Mary's temporal disorientation may have been exacerbated by settling into the respite unit and now preparing to go home again. In these circumstances her agitation may be worsened if she is confronted or corrected. Instead, it is appropriate to reassure her that her daughter is coming directly to the unit and that they will be going home together. Once they get home and Mary settles back into her familiar surroundings, her orientation may well improve. At other times it can be better to simply distract the person or to respond to the emotional content of what they are saying.

> "Isn't it a wonderful summer's day! I want to go out for a walk," Bill says to his daughter, even though it is a cold, dark day in mid-January with snow falling outside. Rather than directly correcting her father, Anne could simply say, "You're in good form today" (responding to the emotional state). "Let's listen to some of your favorite records" (diversion).

To summarize, well-established methods of environmental and behavioral interventions can be readily adapted for use by families. Haley (1983), for example, showed how caregivers can reinforce and cue positive behaviors. Pinkson and Linsk developed an Elderly Support Project where caregivers were trained by supervised social workers to participate in a program of behavioral assessment, development of environmental and behavioral interventions, and nonpharmacological management (Franks 1987).

Environmental Interventions

The foundation of nonpharmacological management is recognizing that the person with dementia is no longer able to adapt, and that instead the environment must be adapted to the patient's specific needs (Knopman and Sawyer-DeMaris 1990). "The ideal environment would be nonstressful, constant, and familiar" (Eimer 1989, p. 434). Studies, however, disagree considerably regarding stimulus reduction, which has been associated with sensory deprivation in the "traditional" long-term care facility, as opposed to stimulus enhancement, which can lead to catastrophic reactions. Further research is required in order to characterize the particular situations where each is appropriate (Berg et al. 1991).

The following suggested interventions apply, to differing extents, in both institutional and home settings (Berg et al. 1991; Chandler 1987; Knopman and Sawyer-DeMaris 1990; Roper et al. 1991; Winograd and Jarvik 1986). Potentially disturbing extraneous stimuli should be minimized by using soft lighting and calm colors such as tan or peach (including the color of uniforms), avoiding abstract or noisy designs, restricting mirrors to dressing areas and bathrooms, using carpets to absorb sound, avoiding loud telephone bells or overhead paging systems, and adding appropriate music but restricting television and radio use. There should be provisions made for safe wandering, with access to the outdoors. Digital keys may be used to allow easy access for cognitively intact persons while restricting those with dementia. Verbal and visual cues should be used together whenever possible. Patients should be allowed to keep familiar possessions, photographs, and mementos and their own clothing. Efforts should be made to include familiar and favorite foods in the diet. With regard to constancy, a regular schedule must be adhered to, families and friends should be discouraged from taking the patient on vacations, and it must be remembered that changing furniture or even adding Christmas decorations can cause confusion and behavioral disturbance.

The environment must also be made safe while allowing patients as much freedom as possible (Chandler 1987; Warshaw 1990). Chairs that recline or swivel should be avoided, and handrails of contrasting color to the walls should be provided. Smoke detectors and fire alarms, in addition to informing neighbors of the situation, may allow patients to remain in their own homes while minimizing the risk of fire. It must be remembered that patients with DAT have difficulty adjusting to new surroundings, and nursing homes report that accidents are most common during the first several weeks of a patient's stay (Warshaw 1990).

Finally, the practice of putting highly agitated patients together in a single unit is not recommended.

Specific Behavioral Interventions

A review of the behavior therapy literature (Wisocki and Mosher 1982) revealed that only 9.6% of research was related to the geriatric population and that of the relevant studies, approximately 75% dealt with institutionalized patients. Institutionalization per se has a number of predictable effects, such as regression, restriction of the behavioral repertoire, social withdrawal, reduced motivation, and increased dependency. Behavior therapy is well suited to this situation, because behavioral interventions are ideal for implementation before maladaptive behaviors develop, and they can continue to have beneficial effects even when staff are not present (Franks 1987).

Despite the finding that in one nursing home survey, chemical and physical restraints were the second and third most commonly used interventions for disruptive behavior, a significant number of staff listed behavioral modification approaches. Of these approaches, 40% used time out (e.g., isolation or leaving the area), 23% used activity diversion (e.g., having patients engage in activities that were incompatible with the disturbed behavior), and 3% used selective reinforcement of desirable behaviors (Whall et al. 1992). In general, however, staff tend to ignore rather than reinforce independent positive behavior and to attend to undesirable behavior such as dependency and agitation. The complexity of the interactions relating to these behaviors makes it necessary to think in terms of the whole institution or family rather than behaviors in isolation (Baltes et al. 1983).

There has been a tendency with dementia patients to work to a model of debility and deterioration. Behavioral therapists have attempted to address this situation by developing a *constructional* approach, which aims to change behavior by concentrating on the adaptive behaviors in the patient's repertoire and increasing the range of behavior. In this approach, efforts are made to channel the person's energy and mobility into more positive activity rather than trying to eliminate unwanted behavior (Brad-bury 1991). A review of the literature on agitation in 1986 (Cohen-Mansfield and Billig 1986) yielded only two studies of behavioral interventions. Mishara and Kastenbaum (1973) demonstrated the effectiveness of an enriched environment and a token economy in self-injurious behavior. Davis (1983) produced a reduction in verbal agitation by combining the reinforcement of incompatible positive behavior with the removal of reinforcement for inappro-priate behavior. The following vignette illustrates some of those techniques.

> Frank, a 68-year-old man with DAT, exhibited the very common symptom of constant calling for his wife and following her ev-erywhere. Eventually she found that she could no longer cope, and Frank was admitted for respite care. On the ward he con-stantly called out and exhibited agitated behavior unless a mem-ber of the staff was with him. Whenever he settled down, the nurse went to attend another patient and the calling started again. At this point a behavioral program was initiated. Only one member of staff on each shift attended to Frank. That nurse sat or walked with him for 10 minutes every half-hour, regardless of his behavior in the meantime, and did not attend him at any other time. Initially he was more agitated; but the reinforcement of negative behavior had been removed, and the stimulus for it (the need for company) was diminished as he received attention on a very regular basis whether he called or not. The program was explained to his wife, and her visits were worked into the schedule. By introducing periods of listening to records he en-joyed and other activities, his wife was able to adapt the program for use at home with some success.

Reminiscence Therapy

Reminiscence involves reliving the past, and for this reason it is a more personal experience than the factual recall of historical events. This form of therapy has become an increasingly popular treatment (Bradbury 1991; Norris 1986). Norris also suggested a number of ways that reminiscence can help patients come to terms with their situation: at least in the early stages of DAT, memory for distant events is relatively preserved compared with recent recall; therefore, reminiscence can be used to maintain self-esteem by focusing on something that the patient can still do. In this way, assets rather than disabilities are highlighted. In addition, reminiscence can help patients to maintain a sense of identity, can allow them to share accumulated experience, and can be an enjoyable activity both for themselves and for younger members of their families.

The evidence for the effectiveness of reminiscence is generally positive though anecdotal. However, for significantly confused or psychotic patients, reminiscence group therapy is less helpful than more structured, less verbally oriented groups and can result in worsening behaviorial disturbance (Lesser et al. 1981). Burnside (1978) found that compared with more highly structured, less verbally oriented groups, reminiscence group therapy was less helpful for significantly confused patients and could result in behavioral disturbance. It is generally agreed, however, that elderly people find reminiscing a comfortable and familiar activity, which can allay their anxiety and defensiveness and over which they can retain control and competence.

Reality Orientation

Reality orientation (RO) was developed in the United States in the 1960s. As defined by the Veterans Administration (Drummond et al. 1978), it is "a basic technique used in the rehabilitation of persons having memory loss, episodes of confusion, and time-place-person disorientation" (Hanley et al. 1981, p. 10). It aims to create an environment that allows patients with memory impairment to function to the limits of their abilities. Two forms of the technique have been described: 24-hour RO and classroom RO.

Classroom RO is an intensive cognitive retraining program held for about 30 minutes each day; 24-hour RO involves active on-ward reorientation throughout the day. There are few empirical data evaluating RO, and it has been the subject of some criticism because of its poor theoretical foundations and questionable relevance to the needs of individual patients (Bradbury 1991; Hanley et al. 1981). Classroom RO has yielded significant relearning in verbal orientation following structured retraining in psychogeriatric populations (Citrin and Dixon 1977; Hanley et al. 1981; Harris and Ivory 1976; Woods 1979). Only Brook et al.

(1975), however, showed any behavioral effects.

Hanley et al. (1981) demonstrated that in contrast to classroom RO, a dramatic improvement in ward orientation behavior could be achieved with 24-hour RO. This suggests that, although both types of RO employ orientation information, behavioral change is not dependent on cognitive change. Rather, the repeated practice of specific behaviors with orientation information cueing, which is reinforced by staff at every opportunity, is the likely mechanism of response (Bradbury 1991; Hanley et al. 1981).

Music Therapy

Music has been recognized as a therapeutic tool with documented psychological and physiological effects, and there has been much anecdotal evidence from families and professionals of the benefits of music for patients with DAT (Glynn 1992). Despite this, little or no empirical research has been done on either the immediate or the long-term effects of music interventions on behavioral symptoms in DAT. Cohen-Mansfield et al. (1990) reported reduced screaming in a study of nursing home residents when there was music in their environment. Cariga et al. (1991) suggested that because vocal agitation serves as a source of self-stimulation for some patients, music interventions could improve behavior by counteracting understimulation. Knopman and Sawyer-DeMaris (1990) found that, in contrast to the often irritating background noise from television, music is usually appreciated and enjoyed by patients with dementia.

Because many elderly patients sway rhythmically, tap their feet, and clap their hands to music with distinct rhythmic patterns, such interventions can be used to increase movement in patients with a limited range of motion. In addition, music interventions can be used in conjunction with reminiscence and reality orientation (Glynn 1992). Finally, it must be remembered—particularly in light of the controversy over stimulus enhancement or reduction—that to optimize the benefits of music interventions, the music must be selected with extreme care (Glynn 1992).

Psychotherapy

Dementia patients are not usually considered for individual psychotherapy because of their poor memory and loss of insight. Psychotherapy, however, can help patients with mild dementia come to terms with their deficits and adjust to their situation (Jeste and Krull 1991). Miller (1989) has demonstrated that many patients are able to deal with emotion-laden issues and can benefit from psychotherapy. There have also been reports of improvement in depressive symptoms in patients with dementia.

Touch

In a survey of nursing management of disruptive behavior, 38% of staff listed touch as an intervention (Whall et al. 1992). The use of touch is not straightforward, however. Birchmore and Clague (1983) and Cariga et al. (1991) reported benefits from tactile stimulation in reducing agitated vocalization, whereas Cohen-Mansfield et al. (1990) found that it increased screaming. Marx et al. (1989), studying the relationship of touch and interpersonal space to agitation, demonstrated divergent responses. Touch was associated with increased aggressive behavior, but touch also decreased physically nonaggressive behaviors, suggesting that in some situations, touch can be a calming form of communication, but in others, it may be misinterpreted and may precipitate aggression and defensiveness.

Approaches for Specific Behavioral Problems

Screaming

Disruptive vocalization tends to occur along with various other agitated behaviors. It has been suggested that it may occur as an atypical feature of depression (Greenwald et al. 1986), but it has also been clearly linked with physical discomfort and with the environment (Cohen-Mansfield et al. 1990). In some cases it tends to occur during patient care activities, particularly toileting and bathing, whereas in other cases it may result from social isolation. Interventions that have been suggested include 1) the use of music (when social isolation and self-stimulation are the problems), 2) a differential reinforcement system rewarding patients for silence or appropriate requests (when screaming is being maintained by contingent staff attention), 3) the use of an audio amplification device allowing the patient's own vocalizations to have an aversive effect (Cariga et al. 1991), 4) the use of operant conditioning techniques (Vaccaro 1988), and possibly 5) the use of touch in selected patients (Birchmore and Clague 1983; Cariga et al. 1991).

Wandering

Rader (1987) has proposed interventions for four categories of wanderers: akathisiacs, modelers, self-stimulators, and exit seekers. Akathisiacs' behavior is often secondary to their medication, which should be reviewed. Modelers follow others around and will stay on the ward as long as the persons they follow do so. Self-stimulators will often go to a door and turn the handle, but not for the purpose of exiting. The exit seekers are trying to leave, although the reason why is often unclear. Surprisingly, wandering has been the subject of very few intervention studies (Dawson and Reid 1987). Two groups reported on the use of protected ward areas for free mobility. Cornbleth (1977) demonstrated that wanderers had a greater range of motion on the ward and nonwanderers had a greater range off the ward. This suggests that the program lifted some restraints from the wanderers but put unnecessary restraints on the nonwanderers. Sawyer and Mendlovitz (1982), who also employed environmental design, reported general satisfaction with the intervention. These interventions and general measures such as the use of identification bracelets, the use of position alarms on the person, putting alarms and complex locks on doors, limiting the amount of cash available, and avoiding restraints should be employed whenever possible (Winograd and Jarvik 1986). As with any behavioral symptom, patients' wandering must first be assessed to exclude pain or any other physical cause (e.g., akathisia secondary to neuroleptics).

The categories of self-stimulator and exit seeker deserve separate discussion. Because the self-stimulator is not trying to exit, the simplest management strategy is to provide alternative forms of stimulation, such as appropriate music or a household task that the person can still accomplish (Hussain and Brown 1987; Rader 1987).

Rader (1987) has described an intervention for exit seekers with the emphasis on allowing as much freedom as possible: because wanderers have a low attention span, distractibility, and impaired memory, the usual group activities are often inappropriate. This can mean that in place of group activities these patients are restrained, with the results that they become even more agitated and their physical strength and balance deteriorate. Therefore, a specifically designed activity program is one of the key aspects of management. In addition, staff should instruct a patient in what staff want the patient to do, rather than what they do not want him or her to do. Negative instruction results in a more complex cognitive process, in which the patient first has to remember the instruction and then has to work out what to do instead. The staff should allow the patient to play out his or her plan, identify a point when he or she might be open to guidance, and then allow the patient to return to the ward without being corrected or confronted.

Many patients with DAT misperceive two-dimensional patterns as barriers. Using this observation, Hussain and Brown (1987) demonstrated that the placement of masking tape in a grid pattern on the floor decreased the frequency of wandering toward exit doors in seven of eight patients. Individuals differed in their responses, however; depending on the pattern used, some patients did not look at the floor, and others were excessively restricted.

Sundown Syndrome and Insomnia

Evans (1987) defined *sundown syndrome* as "the appearance or exacerbation of symptoms of confusion associated with the late afternoon or early evening hours" (p. 101). It is possibly mediated by the abnormalities in the circadian rhythm that are thought to occur in DAT. In support of this possibility, Satlin et al. (1991) reported that the circadian locomotor activity rhythm is disturbed in patients with DAT. Other explanations for sundowning include lack of social contact and the absence of organized activities in the evenings, when nursing home residents are often left alone in their rooms. In fact, studies disagree somewhat about whether the syndrome actually exists. Evans (1987) reported increased agitation in 12.3% of elderly nursing home residents; Cohen-Mansfield et al. (1989) found a more complex relationship, with no clear pattern; and Duggan and McDonald (1992) found no increase in wandering at any time of the day.

In patients with DAT, the normal changes in sleep that occur with aging (reduced REM and slow-wave sleep, with increased wakefulness and daytime napping) are exaggerated (Prinz et al. 1990; Winograd and Jarvik 1986). The management of insomnia and of the postulated sundown syndrome are very similar and are primarily nonpharmacological. At times, both patients and their families have unrealistic expectations about sleep; education may therefore significantly reduce stress without any other intervention (Winograd and Jarvik 1986). As always, physical discomfort and iatrogenic causes must be excluded.

Thereafter, management is aimed at strengthening the normal circadian propensity for sleep and wakefulness by ensuring optimal conditions for daytime activity and nocturnal sleep (sleep hygiene) and by reinforcing normal timegiving cues (zeitgebers) (Gillin and Byerley 1990). Sleep hygiene should be carefully planned by avoiding extremes of temperature, occasional loud noises, illuminated clocks, alcohol (nightcaps), and caffeine. A bedtime snack and regular but not vigorous exercise also promote an appropriate sleep cycle (Swanwick and Clare 1991). Zeitgebers include bright light, social activities, and meals. For instance, appropriately timed bright light can alter the circadian pacemaker and augment its rhythm. Satlin et al. (1992), using this observation, administered evening bright light pulses to patients with DAT and disturbance in the sleep-wake cycle. Although the study was uncontrolled, it suggested that the treatment might improve behavior and sleep in some patients, particularly those with more severe disturbance at baseline. Finally, Okawa et al. (1991) reported improvement in behavior and sleep-wake rhythm in 30% of patients treated by enforcement of social interaction with nurses.

Alcohol and Smoking

The habits of a lifetime are often difficult to break, and both alcohol and smoking present considerable risks to the patient with DAT. With regard to smoking, efforts should be made to persuade the patient to stop. If this is not possible, smoking must be supervised to ensure that the person does not abandon lighted cigarettes. Matches should be kept out of reach, clothes and furniture should be flame resistant wherever possible, smoke detectors/alarms should be installed, and smoking in bed must be banned (Scottish Health Education Group 1988).

The mental effects of alcohol are exaggerated in DAT; even in small amounts, alcohol has the potential to cause disastrous worsening of symptoms. As already mentioned, the practice of giving a nightcap is not recommended. This is not to say that there should always be a total ban on alcohol, but the risks must be considered and each case evaluated individually. Finally, alcohol should not be left where the patient can drink it unsupervised (Scottish Health Education Group 1988).

Driving

Despite their cognitive deficits, a significant number of patients with dementia continue to drive. Waller (1967) found that 31% of drivers in a retirement community had a disorder causing dementia, and O'Neill et al. (1992) reported that almost 20% of dementia patients who attended a memory clinic continued to drive. Patients with DAT can have deficits including memory loss, reduced attention span, disturbance of visual perception, disordered scan paths, reduced visual fields, and poor visuospatial discrimination, any of which may interfere with driving ability (O'Neill 1992b). Patients with DAT were reported to have an accident rate approximately five times that of age-matched control subjects, and almost half have at least one accident before they stop driving (Friedland et al. 1988).

Often family physicians are unaware of their elderly patients' cognitive deficits or driving practice; and to complicate matters further, a significant minority of dementia patients, ranging from 23% (Friedland et al. 1988) to 35% (O'Neill et al. 1992), have been reported to have no deterioration in driving skills. This supports the opinion that a diagnosis of dementia per se should not automatically exclude a person from driving, particularly if other forms of transportation are not readily available. Such a ban could unnecessarily worsen quality of life and result in loss of independence or even institutionalization. A driving history and measurements of activities of daily living appear to be the best available guides, but an on-road driving test appropriate to the person's driving practice is probably the gold standard (O'Neill 1992a). It is clear that doctors should routinely assess their elderly patients' cognitive state and driving practice, that appropriate tests of driving ability need to be developed, and that closer liaison is needed between licensing authorities and the medical profession (O'Neill 1992a).

However, there is no easy, practical way to assess patients, because commonly used psychometric tests do not correlate well with driving ability, driving safety may significantly deteriorate as the disease progresses between assessments, and legal requirements vary widely. In practice, therefore, clinicians should advise that patients stop driving and that alternative forms of transportation be organized as soon as a diagnosis of Alzheimer's disease is made. It must be remembered that even when families together with their physicians make every effort to persuade a patient to stop driving, provide other means of transportation, and ensure that driving licenses and insurance are revoked, some patients will continue to drive. In these circumstances the person's car may have to be disabled.

Incontinence

Urinary and fecal incontinence tend to occur late in the course of dementia. When either develops, the patient must be medically evaluated. If a reversible cause is not found, behavioral interventions and assistance with toileting may be of benefit (Warshaw 1990). With regard to fecal incontinence, placing the patient on the toilet immediately after breakfast will take advantage of the gastrocolic reflex. For urinary incontinence, fluid restriction is not appropriate, and frequent toileting is the treatment of choice.

Restraints can prevent access to appropriate facilities and cause incontinence, particularly at night; they should be avoided whenever possible (Winograd and Jarvik 1986).

Restraints: Use and Abuse

The use of restraints varies widely throughout the United States: 4% of certified nursing homes restrain less than 10% of their residents, but 5% restrain over 90% of their residents (Roper et al. 1991). The overall prevalence of restraint use in long-term care facilities in the United States is estimated to be 41%. In contrast, restraints are much less frequently used in northern Europe (Rader 1991), and Canada is reported to have an eight times greater use than Britain (Brower 1991).

In a survey of nursing attitudes to restraints, most respondents felt that patients should be restrained for safety even if it meant loss of dignity, but the respondents also believed that they themselves should have the right to refuse restraints if they were patients (Scherer et al. 1991). Common reasons for restraints are to prevent wandering, falls, and harm to self or others and to allow provision of medical treatment (e.g., intravenous infusions). There is little evidence, however, that restraints achieve any of these goals. Werner et al. (1989) demonstrated that with restraints, patients continued to have a considerable number of falls, manifested significantly more abnormal movements and vocalizations, and remained agitated. Other reported negative effects of restraint use included skin abrasions and lacerations, urinary incontinence and fecal impaction, contractures and ankylosed joints, demineralization of bone, reduced physical strength and balance, and even death (Brower 1991). Frequently a vicious circle of agitation, restraint, resistance, and increased agitation occurs, which may well end in exhaustion and lethargy (Eigsti and Vrooman 1992). In addition, distress at seeing a person restrained may deter friends or families from visiting and thus result in further isolation and agitation (Brower 1991).

With all these difficulties, it is clearly essential that all staff be trained in the appropriate use of restraints (Stilwell 1991). The dilemma of safety versus autonomy obviously raises ethical (and medicolegal) issues, which have no clearly correct answer and involve strong emotions. Every case must be evaluated on an individual basis, and although the solution may not seem satisfactory to everyone involved, at least a decision should be made in a confident, fair, and dispassionate manner (Hogstel and Gaul 1991). There are alternatives to restraint: the family, environmental, and behavioral interventions already discussed can all be employed to minimize restraint use. Eigsti and Vrooman (1992) demonstrated that a restraint-free policy can result in decreased agitation and increased staff satisfaction. Finally, continuing education, organizational strategies, nursing home design, and nursing philosophies need to be considered if this issue is to be tackled satisfactorily.

Special Care Units

In 1974 the Philadelphia Geriatric Center opened a treatment unit specifically for patients with DAT. Since the 1980s the number of nursing homes with special care units (SCUs) has steadily increased. As already discussed, patients with DAT need special consideration with regard to staffing, environment, security, level of stimulation, activities, and protection from abuse. Traditional nursing homes are often unable to meet these needs, whereas SCUs are specifically designed for the purpose.

A number of issues need to be resolved, however. First, some professionals believe that the possible gains from clustering patients with DAT in single units are outweighed by the absence of role models for adaptive behavior and by the further stigmatization of dementia. In contrast, others believe that there should be even further selection based on the level of impairment; this in turn raises the issue of discharge criteria. Clearly, a patient should remain in the unit as long as he or she benefits from any aspect of the program. A few professionals believe, however, that once admitted, a resident should stay in the unit until death; this practice provides continuity of care for both the patient and the family and also avoids the probable behavioral disturbance that would occur if the patient were discharged (Berg et al. 1991). Finally, despite the considerable cost involved in setting up and staffing SCUs, there are still no definitive studies that demonstrate their efficacy and cost-effectiveness (Berg et al. 1991; Maas 1988).

Conclusions

Although medications may be appropriate for specific behavioral indications, nonpharmacological interventions are the key to management of behavioral disturbance in DAT. Similarly, the hazards of physical restraints generally outweigh any benefits and should be avoided whenever possible. In contrast, the importance of simple measures aimed at avoiding confrontation and maintaining a routine cannot be overemphasized. There is much that families and other nonmedical caregivers can do to help DAT patients without resorting to chemical or physical restraints. This positive trend is reflected in legislation such as the Omnibus Budget Reconciliation Act (1987). There has been surprisingly little research, however, aimed at evaluating specific behavioral, environmental, family, or psychotherapeutic approaches to behavioral disturbances; this research is required if practice is to change.

Despite interest and investment in SCUs, there is little agreement on what constitutes good care for patients with DAT and no clear definition of standard SCU care. Obviously the time is ripe for the regulation of SCUs and research on the benefits of such units. Likewise, the human benefits of managing DAT patients in their own homes through nonpharmacological interventions is obvious, and all such approaches deserve further research and development. There may also, however, be significant economic benefits to such management strategies; this is another area of much-needed study.

References

Alessi CA: Managing the behavioral problems of dementia in the home. Clin Geriatr Med 7:787–801, 1991

Baltes MM, Honn S, Barton EM, et al: On the social ecology of dependence and independence in elderly nursing home residents. J Gerontol 38:556–564, 1983

Beck C, Rossby L, Baldwin B: Correlates of disruptive behavior in cognitively impaired elderly nursing home residents. Arch Psychiatr Nurs 5:281–291, 1991

Berg L, Buchwalter KC, Chafetz PK, et al: Special care units for persons with dementia. J Am Geriatr Soc 39:1229–1236, 1991

Birchmore T, Clague S: A behavioral approach to reduce shouting. Nursing Times 79:37–39, 1983

Bradbury N: Problems of elderly people, in Adult Clinical Problems: A Cognitive Behavioral Approach. Edited by Dryden W, Rentoul R. London, Routledge, 1991, pp 203–231

Brook P, Degun G, Mathew M: Reality orientation, a therapy for psychogeriatric patients: a controlled study. Br J Psychiatry 127:42–45, 1975

Brower HT: The alternatives to restraints. Journal of Gerontological Nursing 17:18–22, 1991

Cariga J, Burgio L, Flynn W, et al: A controlled study of disruptive vocalizations among geriatric residents in nursing homes. J Am Geriatr Soc 39:501–507, 1991

Chandler JD: Geriatric psychiatry. Prim Care 14:761–772, 1987

Citrin CS, Dixon DN: Reality orientation: a milieu therapy used in an institute for the aged. Gerontologist 17:39–43, 1977

Cohen-Mansfield J: Agitated behaviors in the elderly, II: preliminary results in the cognitively deteriorated. J Am Geriatr Soc 34:722–727, 1986

Cohen-Mansfield J, Billig N: Agitated behaviors in the elderly, I: a conceptual review. J Am Geriatr Soc 34:711–721, 1986

Cohen-Mansfield J, Watson V, Meade W: Does sundowning occur in residents of an Alzheimer's unit? International Journal of Geriatric Psychiatry 4:293–298, 1989

Cohen-Mansfield J, Werner P, Marx MS: Screaming in nursing home residents. J Am Geriatr Soc 38:785–792, 1990

Cornbleth T: Effects of a protected hospital ward area on wandering and nonwandering geriatric patients. J Gerontol 32:573–577, 1977

Davis A: Back on their feet: behavioral techniques for elderly patients. Nursing Times 43:26–27, 1983

Dawson P, Reid DW: Behavioral dimensions of patients at risk of wandering. Gerontologist 27:104–107, 1987

Deutsch LH, Rovner BW: Agitation and other non-cognitive abnormalities in Alzheimer's disease. Psychiatr Clin North Am 14:341–351, 1991

Drummond L, Kirchoff L, Scarborough DR: A practical guide to reality orientation. Gerontologist 18:568–573, 1978

Duggan K, McDonald C: Wandering and twilight in a female psychogeriatric population. Psychiatric Bulletin 16:479–481, 1992

Eigsti DG, Vrooman N: Releasing restraints in the nursing home: it can be done. Journal of Gerontological Nursing 18:21–23, 1992

Eimer M: Management of the behavioral symptoms associated with dementia. Prim Care 16:431–450, 1989

Evans LK: Sundown syndrome in the institutionalized elderly. J Am Geriatr Soc 35:101–108, 1987

Franks CM: Behavior therapy and the aging process, in Review of Behavior Therapy: Theory and Practice, Vol 2. Edited by Wilson GT, Franks CM, Kendall PC, et al. New York, Guilford, 1987

Friedland RP, Koss E, Kumar A, et al: Motor vehicle crashes in dementia of the Alzheimer type. Ann Neurol 24:782–786, 1988

Gidley I, Shears R: Alzheimer's: What It Is, How to Cope. London, Unwin Paperbacks, 1988

Gillin JC, Byerley WF: The diagnosis and management of insomnia. N Engl J Med 322:239–248, 1990

Glynn NJ: The music therapy assessment tool in Alzheimer's patients. Journal of Gerontological Nursing 18:3–9, 1992

Greenwald BS, Marin DB, Silverman SM: Serotonergic treatment of screaming and banging in dementia (letter). Lancet 2:1464, 1986

Haley WE: A family approach to the treatment of the cognitively impaired elderly. Gerontologist 23:18–20, 1983

Hanley IG, McGuire RJ, Boyd WD: Reality orientation and dementia: a controlled trial of two approaches. Br J Psychiatry 138:10–14, 1981

Harris CS, Ivory PB: An outcome evaluation of reality orientation therapy with geriatric patients in a state mental hospital. Gerontologist 16:496–504, 1976

Hogstel MO, Gaul AL: Safety or autonomy: an ethical issue for clinical gerontological nursing. Journal of Gerontological Nursing 17:6–11, 1991

Hussain RA, Brown DC: Use of two-dimensional grid patterns to limit hazardous ambulation in demented patients. J Gerontol 42:558–560, 1987

Jeste DV, Krull AJ: Behavioral problems associated with dementia: diagnosis and treatment. Geriatrics 46:28–34, 1991

Knopman DS, Sawyer-DeMaris S: Practical approach to managing behavioral problems in dementia patients. Geriatrics 45:27–35, 1990

Lesser J, Lazarus LW, Frankel R, et al: Reminiscence group therapy with psychotic geriatric inpatients. Gerontologist 21:291–296, 1981

Maas M: Management of patients with Alzheimer's disease in long term care facilities. Nurs Clin North Am 23:57–68, 1988

Mace NL, Rabins PV: The 36 Hour Day. Baltimore, MD, Johns Hopkins University Press, 1981

Marx MS, Werner P, Cohen-Mansfield J: Agitation and touch in the nursing home. Psychol Rep 64:1019–1026, 1989

Miller MD: Opportunities for psychotherapy in the management of dementia. J Geriatr Psychiatry Neurol 2:11–17, 1989

Mishara BL, Kastenbaum R: Self-injurious behavior and environmental change in the institutionalised elderly. Int J Aging Hum Dev 4:133–145, 1973

Murphy E: Dementia and Mental Illness in the Old. New York, Papermac, 1986

New York City Alzheimer's Resource Center: Caring: A Family Guide to Managing the Alzheimer's Patient at Home. New York, New York City Alzheimer's Resource Center, 1985

Norris A: Reminiscence With Elderly People. London, Winslow Press, 1986

Okawa M, Mishima K, Hishikawa Y, et al: Circadian rhythm disorders in sleep–waking and body temperature in elderly patients with dementia and their treatment. Sleep 14:478–485, 1991

O'Neill D: The doctor's dilemma: the ageing driver and dementia. International Journal of Geriatric Psychiatry 7:297–301, 1992a

O'Neill D: Physicians, elderly drivers, and dementia. Lancet 1:41–43, 1992b

O'Neill D, Naubauer K, Boyle M, et al: Dementia and driving. J R Soc Med 85:199–201, 1992

Pillemer K, Moore DW: Abuse of patients in nursing homes: findings from a survey of staff. Gerontologist 29:314–320, 1989

Powell LS, Courtice K: Alzheimer's Disease: A Guide for Families. Reading, MA, Addison-Wesley, 1983

Prinz PN, Vitello MV, Raskind MA, et al: Geriatrics: sleep disorders and aging. N Engl J Med 323:520–526, 1990

Rader J: A comprehensive staff approach to problem wandering. Gerontologist 27:756–760, 1987

Rader J: Modifying the environment to decrease the use of restraints. Journal of Gerontological Nursing 17:9–13, 1991

Reisberg B: A Guide to Alzheimer's Disease: For Families, Spouses, and Friends. New York, Collier Macmillan, 1983

Roper JM, Shapira J, Chang BL: Agitation in the demented patient: a framework for management. Journal of Gerontological Nursing 17:17–21, 1991

Rovner BW, Edelman BA, Cox MP, et al: The impact of antipsychotic drug regulations on psychotropic prescribing practices in nursing homes. Am J Psychiatry 149:1390–1392, 1992

Satlin A, Teicher MH, Lieberman HR, et al: Circadian locomotor activity rhythms in Alzheimer's disease. Neuropsychopharmacology 5:115–126, 1991

Satlin A, Volicer L, Ross V, et al: Bright light treatment of behavioral and sleep disturbances in patients with Alzheimer's disease. Am J Psychiatry 149:1028–1032, 1992

Sawyer JC, Mendlovitz AA: A management program for ambulatory institutionalized patients with Alzheimer's disease and related disorders. Paper presented at the annual conference of the Gerontological Society, Boston, MA, November 1982

Scherer YK, Janelli LM, Kanski GW: The nursing dilemma of restraints. Journal of Gerontological Nursing 17:14–17, 1991

Scottish Health Education Group: Coping With Dementia: A Handbook for Carers. Edinburgh, UK, Scottish Health Education Group, p 62

Stilwell EM: Are nurses educated on the use of restraints? Journal of Gerontological Nursing 17:23–26, 1991

Swanwick GRJ, Clare AW: The management of insomnia. Journal of the Irish Colleges of Physicians and Surgeons 20:249–250, 1991

Teri L, Logsdon R: Assessment and management of behavioral disturbances in Alzheimer's disease. Compr Ther 16:36–42, 1990

Teri L, Larson EB, Reifler BV: Behavioral disturbance in dementia of the Alzheimer's type. J Am Geriatr Soc 36:1–6, 1988

Thomas DR: Assessment and management of agitation in the elderly. Geriatrics 43:45–53, 1988

Vaccaro FJ: Successful operant conditioning procedures with an institutionalised aggressive geriatric patient. Int J Aging Hum Dev 26:71–79, 1988

Waller JA: Cardiovascular disease, aging, and traffic accidents. Journal of Chronic Disease 20:615–620, 1967

Warshaw GA: New perspectives in the management of Alzheimer's disease. Am Fam Physician 42:41S–47S (November), 1990

Watt J, Calder A: I Love You But You Drive Me Crazy. Vancouver, Forbes Publications, 1981

Werner P, Cohen-Mansfield J, Braun J, et al: Physical restraints and agitation in nursing home residents. J Am Geriatr Soc 37:1122–1126, 1989

Whall AL, Gillis GL, Yankou D, et al: Disruptive behavior in elderly nursing home residents: a survey of nursing staff. Journal of Gerontological Nursing 18:13–17, 1992

Wilcock G: Living With Alzheimer's Disease. Harmondsworth, UK, Penguin, 1990

Winograd CH, Jarvik LF: Physician management of the demented patient. J Am Geriatr Soc 34:295–308, 1986

Wisocki PA, Mosher P: The elderly: an understudied population in behavioral research. International Journal of Behavioral Geriatrics 1:5–14, 1982

Woods RT: Alzheimer's Disease: Coping With a Living Death. London, Souvenir Press, 1989

Woods RT: Reality orientation and staff attention: a controlled study. Br J Psychiatry 134:502–507, 1979

Wragg RE, Jeste DV: Neuroleptics and alternative treatments: management of behavioral symptoms and psychosis in Alzheimer's disease and related conditions. Psychiatr Clin North Am 11:195–213, 1988

CHAPTER 11

Pharmacotherapy of Behavioral Symptoms in Dementia: Nonneuroleptic Agents

Alan M. Mellow, M.D., Ph.D.
Stephen M. Aronson, M.D.

*T*he behavioral complications of Alzheimer's disease and other dementias are responsible for much of the suffering, family disruption, and economic hardship that characterize the devastating course of these disorders (Burns et al. 1990; Deutsch and Rovner 1991). Agitation, aggression, and wandering are seen in at least 75% of patients with Alzheimer's disease, and symptoms of frank psychosis occur at some point in the course of illness in at least 50% (Reisberg et al. 1987; Wragg and Jeste 1989). Furthermore, patients with psychosis may represent a subgroup with a more rapid progression of the dementia syndrome (Drevets and Rubin 1989; Rosen and Zubenko 1991). It is clear that, even in the absence of definitive treatment for the cognitive impairment seen in Alzheimer's disease and other dementias, alleviation of some behavioral complications can often improve the quality of life and decrease the stress on patients and caregivers.

A variety of behavioral manipulations have been reported as being useful in the management of dementia patients (Chrisman et al. 1991; Maletta 1988; Roper et al. 1991). Many patients, however, require pharmacological treatment. The mainstay of this pharmacotherapy has for years been the judicious use of neuro-leptic agents (Devanand et al. 1989; Raskind et al. 1987; Risse and Barnes 1986). This approach is limited by both the low efficacy of these agents and their significant side effects (Schneider et al. 1990; Wragg and Jeste 1988). Consequently, there is now consid-erable interest in the use of nonneuroleptic psychopharmacologi-cal agents in the management of behavioral disturbance in Alzheimer's disease and other dementias (Schneider and Sobin 1992). In this chapter we review what is known of the clinical use of nonneuroleptic agents in the management of the behavioral complications of dementia, with a special emphasis on a rationale for clinical trials and methodological issues.

Rationale for Nonneuroleptic Therapy—A Search for Mechanisms?

The imperative of the demands that agitated dementia patients place on the health care system provides the empirical rationale for developing safe, effective treatments for these patients. The goal, however, is someday to provide treatment based on the underlying pathophysiology. Although the current state of the art does not allow for such a mechanism-based therapeutic ap-proach, some work has attempted to characterize specific neuro-chemical features associated with disturbed behavior in dementia (Dursun 1992; Schneider et al. 1988; Zubenko et al. 1991). Optimal therapies should ultimately be based on such findings. As is seen from what follows, the current rationale for many of these interventions is often based on "antiaggressivity" properties of the relevant agents, either in animal studies or in other clinical populations.

Drugs Used for Disturbed Behavior in Alzheimer's and Other Dementias

Beta-Blocking Agents

Beta-adrenergic blocking agents, particularly propranolol, have been used clinically for many years in the management of agita-

tion and self-injurious behavior in patients with mental retardation (Ratey et al. 1986; Ruedrich et al. 1990). In the past decade,
patients with agitation and assaultiveness in the context of a
variety of organic brain syndromes (largely not Alzheimer's disease) have been treated with beta-blockers in open trials, with
modest improvements in disturbed behavior (Greendyke et al.
1984; Yudofsky et al. 1981). Only two studies have specifically
addressed agitated patients with dementia (Petrie and Ban 1981;
Weiler et al. 1988). Again, these were uncontrolled, but they
showed some benefits with propranolol treatment. Greendyke et
al. (1986) have conducted several placebo-controlled trials with
both propranolol and the nonselective beta-adrenergic blocker
pindolol (Greendyke and Kanter 1986; Greendyke et al. 1989).
These studies, again involving patients without the diagnosis of
Alzheimer's disease, demonstrated significant improvements in
behavior.

Thus, the bulk of the published evidence for the use of beta-
blocking agents in the management of agitated behaviors does
not include patients with primary dementia. Controlled trials are
therefore needed. One limitation of this approach in treating
elderly dementia patients is the attendant contraindications (dia-
betes, congestive heart failure, chronic obstructive pulmonary
disease) and side effects (hypotension, bradycardia, confusion) of
beta-blocking agents in this population, particularly because the
doses required for clinical effect may be quite high (up to 560
mg/day in several studies). From the standpoint of mechanism,
although noradrenergic mechanisms have been proposed to be
involved in agitated states in patients with depression (Mann et
al. 1985), neurochemical evidence in postmortem studies in Alzheimer's disease patients indicates a preservation of brain norepinephrine in association with psychosis (Zubenko et al. 1991).
Thus the utility, both from a clinical and a theoretical standpoint,
of a beta-blocker strategy in disruptive behaviors in Alzheimer's
disease and other dementias remains unclear.

Lithium

In addition to its well-known use in the treatment of mood
disorders, lithium has long been suggested as an agent with

"antiaggressivity" properties in humans, even in subjects without psychotic or mood disorders (Sheard et al. 1976). Like beta-blockers, lithium has been used clinically for aggressive behavior in patients with brain injury (Glenn et al. 1989) and mental retardation (Spreat et al. 1989). Published experience with dementia patients is, however, quite limited. In an open trial of 10 patients with mixed organic brain syndrome diagnoses, but including alcoholism and affective symptomatology, Williams and Goldstein (1979) reported improvement in agitation and sleep disturbance in 6 of 8 patients, with a mean lithium carbonate dose of 1200 mg/day. Another open trial reported significant toxicity and no therapeutic effect in a group of elderly patients with mixed chronic brain syndrome diagnoses. In the only published clinical series reported in which patients with Alzheimer's disease were studied exclusively (Randels et al. 1984), only 2 of 9 patients had improvement in agitated behavior. Finally, 2 cases were reported (Essa 1986; Havens and Cole 1982) of behavioral improvement after lithium treatment in dementia, but with significant toxicity in the latter case. In summary, there are few controlled data to support the efficacy of lithium in the treatment of behavioral disturbance in primary dementia. A well-designed controlled trial has not been performed; toxicity may be limiting in many Alzheimer's disease patients.

Serotonergic Agents

Because there is considerable evidence linking the neurotransmitter serotonin (5-HT) to aggression and impulsivity (Coccaro 1989; Linnoila and Virkkunen 1992), agents affecting 5-HT might be candidates for treating aggressive behavior in dementia. The first of these was the sedating antidepressant trazodone, which has mixed properties of 5-HT agonist and antagonist and uptake inhibition. Nair et al. (1973) reported behavioral improvement in 8 of 10 dementia patients receiving trazodone up to 150 mg/day. Subsequent case reports (Greenwald et al. 1986; Tingle 1986) and open series (Gedye 1991; Pinner and Rich 1988; Simpson and Foster 1986) in patients with mixed dementia diagnoses reported improvement in up to half the patients studied, in dosages up to 500 mg/day. A recent placebo-controlled study with trazodone in

Alzheimer's disease demonstrated a small but significant improvement in behavioral symptoms (Lawlor et al. 1994). Trazodone may have some promise, but again, further controlled trials are needed.

Selective serotonin reuptake inhibitors (SSRIs) have been another approach to this problem. In an open study, Bergman et al. (1983) reported behavioral improvement in 5 of 12 Alzheimer's disease patients treated with the SSRI alaproclate. A subsequent controlled trial failed to show any efficacy (Dehlin et al. 1985). In a large, controlled multicenter study (Nyth and Gottfries 1990), citalopram produced behavioral improvement, including improvement in affective symptoms, making it possible that the observed benefit was related to the antidepressant properties of the drug. Finally, fluoxetine was reported as effective in a case report of agitation in posttraumatic dementia (Sobin et al. 1989).

Several studies have reported the use of serotonin agonists. A number of case reports (Colenda 1988; Tiller et al. 1988) and one recent open study (Sakauye et al. 1993) showed behavioral improvement following buspirone, a novel anxiolytic with 5-HT_{1a} agonist properties. In a placebo-controlled trial with the 5-HT_1 agonist m-chlorophenylpiperazine (m-CPP), a trazodone metabolite, no behavioral improvement was noted (Lawlor et al. 1991).

In summary, serotonergic interventions, for which there may be a neurochemical rationale, require more study in this population.

Benzodiazepines

Although clinical wisdom teaches that patients with dementia are particularly sensitive to the adverse effects of benzodiazepines, early studies (Beber 1965; Chesrow 1965; Gerz 1964) reported some efficacy for oxazepam in reducing agitation in a mixed elderly "brain disease" population. This suggests that future trials with low-dose, short-acting benzodiazepines in patients with well-diagnosed Alzheimer's disease or other dementia might be warranted (Stern et al. 1991).

L-Deprenyl (Selegiline)

Since the observations of increased activity of brain monoamine oxidase type B (MAO-B) in aging and Alzheimer's disease (Oreland and Gottfries 1986; Sparks et al. 1991), there has been considerable interest in the use of the selective MAO-B inhibitor L-deprenyl in low doses in the treatment of both cognitive and noncognitive symptoms in Alzheimer's disease. In open trials with inpatients with both Alzheimer's disease and multi-infarct dementia (MID) (Martini et al. 1987) and with Alzheimer's disease outpatients (Schneider et al. 1991), treatment with L-deprenyl resulted in general behavioral improvement. Five of eight Alzheimer's disease patients with severe dementia showed improvement in a single-blind study (Goad et al. 1991). Results of double-blind, placebo-controlled trials have been conflicting, showing both mild improvement (Tariot et al. 1987) and no improvement (Burke et al. 1993).

Anticonvulsants

A promising area of research has been the use of anticonvulsants (particularly those effective in treating mood disorders) in the management of behavioral symptoms in dementia. Carbamazepine has long been proposed as a treatment for aggressive behavior in patients with brain damage of various types (Foster et al. 1989; Garbutt and Loosen 1983; Lewin and Sumners 1992). Several case reports have demonstrated significant improvement with carbamazepine treatment in severe behavioral disturbance in dementia patients (Essa 1986; Leibovici and Tariot 1988; Marin and Greenwald 1989). The use of carbamazepine has more recently been extended to two small open trials (Gleason and Schneider 1990; Patterson 1988). One double-blind trial (Chambers et al. 1982) failed to detect improvement, but the carbamazepine doses used achieved relatively low plasma levels. In our own retrospective study (A. M. Mellow and S. M. Aronson, unpublished data, May 1991) of 31 chronic inpatients with various dementia diagnoses, two-thirds of the patients were rated as behaviorally improved. A recent pilot placebo-controlled study with carbamazepine demonstrated a reduction in agitated behaviors in dementia patients (Tariot et al. 1994). Although larger, controlled clinical trials are needed, carbamazepine may be considered a potentially useful addition to the armamentarium of agents in this arena.

Sodium valproate is another anticonvulsant with antimanic properties (Pope et al. 1991) that has been reported to have antiaggressivity effects in animal models (Puglisi et al. 1981; Simler et al. 1983) and might be of use in dementia. We found marked or moderate improvement in behavior in three of four patients with severe dementia after valproate treatment (Mellow et al. 1993). This finding must be confirmed by larger series and controlled trials.

Summary and Conclusions

As the population ages and the overall prevalence of dementia dramatically increases over the next few decades, the clinical problem of disturbed behavior as a complication of dementia will take center stage as a major public health issue. The personal and economic toll of dementia could be lessened by reducing the need for hospitalization and delaying expensive nursing home placement. Hence, the search for safe, effective treatments for these behaviors must be a priority. As is clear from this review, that search is still in its infancy. What is also clear from the published literature is the pressing need for rigorously designed, placebo-controlled clinical trials with well-validated outcome measures to confirm and extend the available preliminary findings, particularly those with serotonergic and anticonvulsant agents. In addition, although many disturbed behaviors may transcend several dementia diagnoses, studies with homogeneous patient samples are required. Finally, correlations of patients' clinical and biological features with their treatment response to selected agents would not only provide critical, clinically useful information, but might also shed light on the biochemical underpinnings of agitation and other behavioral disturbances in dementia.

References

Beber CR: Management of behavior in the institutionalized aged. Diseases of the Nervous System 26:591–595, 1965

Bergman I, Brane G, Gottfries CG, et al: Alaproclate: a pharmacokinetic and biochemical study in patients with dementia of Alzheimer type. Psychopharmacology (Berl) 80:279–283, 1983

Burke WJ, Ranno AE, Roccaforte WH, et al: L-Deprenyl in the treatment of mild dementia of the Alzheimer type: preliminary results. J Am Geriatr Soc 41:367–370, 1993

Burns A, Jacoby R, Levy R: Psychiatric phenomena in Alzheimer's disease, IV: disorders of behaviour. Br J Psychiatry 157:86–94, 1990

Chambers CA, Bain J, Rosbottom R, et al: Carbamazepine in senile dementia and overactivity—a placebo controlled double blind trial. International Research Communications System Journal of Medical Science 10:505–506, 1982

Chesrow EJ: Blind study of oxazepam in the management of geriatric patients with behavioral problems. Clinical Medicine 72:1001–1005, 1965

Chrisman M, Tabar D, Whall AL, et al: Agitated behavior in the cognitively impaired elderly. Journal of Gerontological Nursing 17:9–13, 1991

Coccaro EF: Central serotonin and impulsive aggression. Br J Psychiatry Suppl 8:52–62, 1989

Colenda CC: Buspirone in treatment of agitated dementia patient (letter). Lancet 2:1169, 1988

Dehlin O, Hedenrud B, Jansson P, et al: A double-blind comparison of alaproclate and placebo in the treatment of patients with senile dementia. Acta Psychiatr Scand 71:190–196, 1985

Deutsch LH, Rovner BW: Agitation and other noncognitive abnormalities in Alzheimer's disease. Psychiatr Clin North Am 14:341–351, 1991

Devanand DP, Sackeim HA, Brown RP, et al: A pilot study of haloperidol treatment of psychosis and behavioral disturbance in Alzheimer's disease. Arch Neurol 46:854–857, 1989

Drevets WC, Rubin EH: Psychotic symptoms and the longitudinal course of senile dementia of the Alzheimer type. Biol Psychiatry 25:39–48, 1989

Dursun SM: 5-HT$_2$ receptors, hallucinations, and dementia (letter). Br J Psychiatry 161:719, 1992

Essa M: Carbamazepine in dementia. J Clin Psychopharmacol 6:234–236, 1986

Foster HG, Hillbrand M, Chi CC: Efficacy of carbamazepine in assaultive patients with frontal lobe dysfunction. Prog Neuropsychopharmacol Biol Psychiatry 13:865–874, 1989

Garbutt JC, Loosen PT: Is carbamazepine helpful in paroxysmal behavior disorders? Am J Psychiatry 140:1363–1364, 1983

Gedye A: Serotonergic treatment for aggression in a Down's syndrome adult showing signs of Alzheimer's disease. Journal of Mental Deficiency Research 5:247–258, 1991

Gerz H: A preliminary report on the management of geriatric patients with oxazepam. Am J Psychiatry 120:1110–1111, 1964

Gleason RP, Schneider LS: Carbamazepine treatment of agitation in Alzheimer's outpatients refractory to neuroleptics. J Clin Psychiatry 51:115–118, 1990

Glenn MB, Wroblewski B, Parziale J, et al: Lithium carbonate for aggressive behavior or affective instability in ten brain-injured patients. Am J Phys Med Rehabil 68:221–226, 1989

Goad DL, Davis CM, Liem P, et al: The use of selegiline in Alzheimer's patients with behavior problems. J Clin Psychiatry 52:342–345, 1991

Greendyke RM, Kanter DR: Therapeutic effects of pindolol on behavioral disturbances associated with organic brain disease: a double blind study. J Clin Psychiatry 47:423–426, 1986

Greendyke RM, Schuster DB, Wooton JA: Propranolol in the treatment of assaultive patients with organic brain disease. J Clin Psychopharmacol 4:282–285, 1984

Greendyke RM, Kanter DR, Schuster DB, et al: Propranolol treatment of assaultive patients with organic brain disease: a double-blind crossover, placebo-controlled study. J Nerv Ment Dis 174:290–294, 1986

Greendyke RM, Berkner JP, Webster JC, et al: Treatment of behavioral problems with pindolol. Psychosomatics 30:161–165, 1989

Greenwald BS, Marin DB, Silverman SM: Serotoninergic treatment of screaming and banging in dementia. Lancet 2:1464–1465, 1986

Havens WW, Cole J: Successful treatment of dementia with lithium (letter). J Clin Psychopharmacol 2:71–72, 1982

Lawlor BA, Sunderland T, Mellow AM, et al: A pilot placebo-controlled study of chronic m-CPP administration in Alzheimer's disease. Biol Psychiatry 30:140–144, 1991

Lawlor BA, Radcliffe J, Molchan SE, et al: A pilot placebo-controlled study of trazodone and buspirone in Alzheimer's disease. International Journal of Geriatric Psychiatry 9:55–59, 1994

Leibovici A, Tariot PN: Carbamazepine treatment of agitation associated with dementia. J Geriatr Psychiatry Neurol 1:110–112, 1988

Lewin J, Sumners D: Successful treatment of episodic dyscontrol with carbamazepine. Br J Psychiatry 161:261–262, 1992

Linnoila VM, Virkkunen M: Aggression, suicidality, and serotonin. J Clin Psychiatry 53:46–51, 1992

Maletta GJ: Management of behavior problems in elderly patients with Alzheimer's disease and other dementias. Clin Geriatr Med 4:719–747, 1988

Mann JJ, Brown RP, Halper JP, et al: Reduced sensitivity of lymphocyte beta-adrenergic receptors in patients with endogenous depression and psychomotor agitation. N Engl J Med 313:715–720, 1985

Marin DB, Greenwald BS: Carbamazepine for aggressive agitation in demented patients during nursing care (letter). Am J Psychiatry 146:805, 1989

Martini E, Pataky I, Szilagyi K, et al: Brief information on an early phase-II study with deprenyl in demented patients. Pharmacopsychiatry 20:256–257, 1987

Mellow AM, Solano-Lopez C, Davis S: Sodium valproate in the treatment of behavioral disturbance in dementia. J Geriatr Psychiatry Neurol 6:205–209, 1993

Nair NP, Ban TA, Hontela S, et al: Trazodone in the treatment of organic brain syndromes, with special reference to psychogeriatrics. Current Therapeutic Research: Clinical and Experimental 15:769–775, 1973

Nyth AL, Gottfries CG: The clinical efficacy of citalopram in treatment of emotional disturbances in dementia disorders: a Nordic multicentre study. Br J Psychiatry 157:894–901, 1990

Oreland L, Gottfries CG: Brain and brain monoamine oxidase in aging and in dementia of Alzheimer's type. Prog Neuropsychopharmacol Biol Psychiatry 10:533–540, 1986

Patterson JF: A preliminary study of carbamazepine in the treatment of assaultive patients with dementia. J Geriatr Psychiatry Neurol 1:21–23, 1988

Petrie WM, Ban TA: Propranolol in organic agitation (letter). Lancet 1:324, 1981

Pinner E, Rich CL: Effects of trazodone on aggressive behavior in seven patients with organic mental disorders. Am J Psychiatry 145:1295–1296, 1988

Pope HG, McElroy SL, Keck PJ, et al: Valproate in the treatment of acute mania: a placebo-controlled study. Arch Gen Psychiatry 48:62–68, 1991

Puglisi AS, Simler S, Kempf E, et al: Involvement of the GABAergic system on shock-induced aggressive behavior in two strains of mice. Pharmacol Biochem Behav 1:13–18, 1981

Randels PM, Marco LA, Ford DI, et al: Lithium and lecithin treatment in Alzheimer's disease: a pilot study. Hillside Journal of Clinical Psychiatry 6:139–147, 1984

Raskind MA, Risse SC, Lampe TH: Dementia and antipsychotic drugs. J Clin Psychiatry 48 (suppl):16–18, 1987

Ratey JJ, Mikkelsen EJ, Smith GB, et al: Beta-blockers in the severely and profoundly mentally retarded. J Clin Psychopharmacol 6:103–107, 1986

Reisberg B, Borenstein J, Salob SP, et al: Behavioral symptoms in Alzheimer's disease: phenomenology and treatment. J Clin Psychiatry 48:9–15, 1987

Risse SC, Barnes R: Pharmacologic treatment of agitation associated with dementia. J Am Geriatr Soc 34:368–376, 1986

Roper JM, Shapira J, Chang BL: Agitation in the demented patient: a framework for management. Journal of Gerontological Nursing 17:17–21, 1991

Rosen J, Zubenko GS: Emergence of psychosis and depression in the longitudinal evaluation of Alzheimer's disease. Biol Psychiatry 29:224–232, 1991

Ruedrich SL, Grush L, Wilson J: Beta adrenergic blocking medications for aggressive or self-injurious mentally retarded persons. Am J Ment Retard 95:110–119, 1990

Sakauye KM, Camp CJ, Ford PA: Effects of buspirone on agitation associated with dementia. American Journal of Geriatric Psychiatry 1:82–84, 1993

Schneider LS, Sobin PS: Non-neuroleptic treatment of behavioral symptoms and agitation in Alzheimer's disease and other dementias. Psychopharmacol Bull 28:71–79, 1992

Schneider LS, Severson JA, Chui HC, et al: Platelet tritiated imipramine binding and MAO activity in Alzheimer's disease patients with agitation and delusions. Psychiatry Res 25:311–322, 1988

Schneider LS, Pollock VE, Lyness SA: A metaanalysis of controlled trials of neuroleptic treatment in dementia. J Am Geriatr Soc 38:553–563, 1990

Schneider LS, Pollock VE, Zemansky MF, et al: A pilot study of low-dose L-deprenyl in Alzheimer's disease. J Geriatr Psychiatry Neurol 4:143–148, 1991

Sheard MH, Marini JL, Bridges CI, et al: The effect of lithium on impulsive aggressive behavior in man. Am J Psychiatry 1133:1409–1413, 1976

Simler S, Puglisi AS, Mandel P: Effects of n-di-propylacetate on aggressive behavior and brain GABA level in isolated mice. Pharmacol Biochem Behav 18:717–720, 1983

Simpson DM, Foster D: Improvement in organically disturbed behavior with trazodone treatment. J Clin Psychiatry 47:191–193, 1986

Sobin P, Schneider L, McDermott H: Fluoxetine in the treatment of agitated dementia (letter). Am J Psychiatry 146:1636, 1989

Sparks DL, Woeltz VM, Markesbery WR: Alterations in brain monoamine oxidase activity in aging, Alzheimer's disease and Pick's disease. Arch Neurol 48:718–721, 1991

Spreat S, Behar D, Reneski B, et al: Lithium carbonate for aggression in mentally retarded persons. Compr Psychiatry 30:505–511, 1989

Stern RG, Duffelmeyer ME, Zemishlani Z, et al: The use of benzodiazepines in the management of behavioral symptoms in demented patients. Psychiatr Clin North Am 14:375–384, 1991

Tariot PN, Cohen RM, Sunderland T, et al: L-deprenyl in Alzheimer's disease: preliminary evidence for behavioral change with monoamine oxidase B inhibition. Arch Gen Psychiatry 44:427–433, 1987

Tariot PN, Erb R, Leibovici A, et al:Carbamazepine treatment of agitation in ursing home patients with dementia: a preliminary study. J Am Geriatr Soc 42:1160–1166, 1994

Tiller JWG, Dakis JA, Shaw JM: Short-term buspirone treatment in disinhibition with dementia (letter). Lancet 2:510, 1988

Tingle D: Trazodone in dementia (letter). J Clin Psychiatry 47:482, 1986

Weiler PG, Mungas D, Bernick C: Propranolol for the control of disruptive behavior in senile dementia. J Geriatr Psychiatry Neurol 1:226–230, 1988

Williams KH, Goldstein G: Cognitive and affective responses to lithium in patients with organic brain syndrome. Am J Psychiatry 136:800–803, 1979

Wragg RE, Jeste DV: Neuroleptics and alternative treatments: management of behavioral symptoms and psychosis in Alzheimer's disease and related conditions. Psychiatr Clin North Am 11:195–213, 1988

Wragg RE, Jeste DV: Overview of depression and psychosis in Alzheimer's disease. Am J Psychiatry 146:577–587, 1989

Yudofsky S, Williams D, Gorman J: Propranolol in the treatment of rage and violent behavior in patients. Am J Psychiatry 138:218–220, 1981

Zubenko GS, Moossy J, Martinez AJ, et al: Neuropathologic and neurochemical correlates of psychosis in primary dementia. Arch Neurol 48:619–624, 1991

Section IV

Psychosocial Impact

CHAPTER 12

Caregiver Distress and Behavioral Symptoms

Carol Magai, Ph.D.
Renata Hartung, B.A.
Carl I. Cohen, M.D.

*N*othing in life prepares a person to face the discovery that a loved one is afflicted with Alzheimer's disease. The gradual onset and slow progress of the disease, along with the human tendency to deny unpleasant realizations, often causes relatives to avoid, for as long as possible, putting their fears and suspicions to the test by seeking professional consultation. When the diagnosis is finally made, family members experience a range of emotions—from relief at getting clarity to fear and despair as they anticipate a grim future. Emotional stress continues for those who bear the primary burden of care over the long course of the illness as they must confront alterations in personality, cognition, and behavior.

Caregivers are at high risk for developing psychological distress (George and Gwyther 1984; Whitlatch et al. 1991). For example, the incidence of depression in adult caregivers of dementia patients has ranged from 14% to 47% in various samples (see review by Dura et al. 1991). An additional 10% of caregivers have been found to meet DSM-III-R criteria for anxiety (Dura et al.

The authors thank Carole Lefkowitz for her assistance. The work was supported in part by Grant P30AG08051 from the National Institute on Aging.

1991). Anger and resentment are other emotions commonly felt during the caregiving experience. Such feelings sometimes border on violence. In a study of 236 family caregivers of dementia patients, Pillemer and Suitor (1992) found that one-fifth experienced violent feelings and feared they might act on their impulses. Of that one-fifth, one-third reported that they had actually engaged in violent behavior.

Caregiver distress is also one of the most important predictors of the decision to institutionalize a family member (Brown et al. 1990; Townsend 1990). Ferris and associates (1987) found that one-third of the spouses and one-sixth of the children of Alzheimer's disease patients had some kind of emotional complaint before placement of their relative in a nursing home, mainly depression in spouses and anxiety in children. In terms of patient characteristics before institutionalization, the chief factors in precipitating placement in a nursing home were agitation and violence, incontinence, and wandering (Ferris et al. 1987). However, caregiver emotional distress may not be alleviated after the patient is institutionalized. The caregiver's stress may be responsible for the institutionalization, but the act itself introduces its own traumatic stress, inducing feelings of helplessness and guilt and the threat of financial ruin, especially in middle-class families, who cannot have Medicaid assistance.

Although it is evident that caregiving has enormous psychological impact, it is less certain which elements of the caregiving experience contribute to or mitigate this distress. Such information could greatly enhance treatment strategies and assist policy makers. In this chapter we focus our attention on the effects of patient behavior—generally recognized as one of the most potent stressors in dementia—on caregiver distress, on what factors exacerbate and modulate the impact of behavioral symptoms, and on whether there are interventions that can modify its harmful consequences.

Conceptual Issues

Understanding the impact of the behavior of Alzheimer's disease patients on their caregivers is heavily dependent on concepts of *behavior* and *impact.* Although behavior is addressed in greater detail elsewhere in this volume, it is essential to recognize that *behavior* has been variously defined in the literature to include virtually all cognitive, behavioral, and emotional responses to the patient (Alessi 1991); to exclude cognitive disturbances but to include behavioral and emotional elements (Pearlin et al. 1990; Teresi et al. 1988–1989); or to be limited to certain circumscribed areas such as activities of daily living (Zarit 1989) or aggressivity (Cohen-Mansfield et al. 1989, 1990). In our discussion, we have generally excluded cognitive dimensions from our concept of behavior. Consequently, it was often necessary for us to dissect behavioral components from the more general categories used in many studies.

Likewise, concepts of impact on caregivers have varied widely. Table 12–1 provides an overview of the more frequently employed measures of impact. Some theorists have viewed impact as primarily a subjective response, whereas others have focused on its objective qualities. Moreover, subjective impacts have been subdivided into emotional (e.g., depression) and cognitive (e.g., helplessness) responses, and objective impacts have been subdivided into behavioral (e.g., tasks) and cognitive (e.g., inconvenience) elements.

Our discussion is further complicated by the fact that patients' behavioral symptoms change over the course of the illness, which is nevertheless characterized by an ineluctable decline in cognitive functioning (Haley and Pardo 1989). Caregivers' reactions have been typically addressed within the framework of three theories (Haley and Pardo 1989): 1) the wear-and-tear hypothesis, which proposes that there is a progressive deterioration of both patient and caregiver as the dementia progresses and the caregiver is burdened with more and more stressors; 2) the adaptational hypothesis, which proposes that the caregiver either stabilizes or improves over time; and 3) the trait hypothesis, which maintains that adaptational level remains constant over the course of the disease because of stable personality dispositions and coping styles. Unfortunately, none of these models takes into account the fact that whereas cognitive abilities decline steadily, behavioral problems tend to emerge, peak, and recede, only to be replaced with others.

The impact of behaviors has also been confounded by the effects of the caregivers' gender, age, relationship, class, and ethnicity. Female caregivers typically experience more burden than their male counterparts (Barusch and Spaid 1989; Borden and Berlin 1990; Cantor 1983; Coward and Dwyer 1990; Fitting et

Table 12–1.   Terminology used to examine impact of stressors on caregiving

Consequences for caregiver	Description
Psychological well-being	Measures of positive and negative emotions (e.g., depression, anxiety) (George and Gwyther 1986; Lawton 1984)
Subjective burden	Emotional responses to demands of caregiving (Montgomery et al. 1985)
Objective burden	Actual demands on caregiver time and resources (Montgomery et al. 1985)
Burden	Perceived impact of caregiving on several domains such as physical and emotional well-being, personal activities, family life, and finances (Zarit et al. 1986)
Impact	Negative charges in caregiver's relationships and activities (Poulshock and Deimling 1984)
Strain	Manifestations of burden such as psychological disturbance, reduction of social activities, and feelings of hopelessness (Morycz 1985)
Inconvenience	The degree to which caregiving has altered time for recreation, financial situation, work performance, and health (Wilder et al. 1983)
Distress	Biopsychosocial responses to stressors as well as to moderating factors such as vulnerability (e.g., health, demographic variables) and personal resources (e.g., coping, social networks) (Vitaliano et al. 1989)
Hassles and uplifts	Small, daily stressors (hassles) and small satisfactions (uplifts) experienced by caregiver (Kinney and Stephens 1989)
Reaction	Degree to which individual patient behaviors bother or upset the caregiver (Teri et al. 1992)

al. 1986; Horowitz 1985; Parks and Pilisuk 1991; Zarit et al. 1983). This finding appears to be independent of demographic and socioeconomic variables and relationship to care receivers. A recent metanalysis by Miller and Cafasso (1992) estimated that female caregivers are 20% more burdened than male caregivers.

Although caregiving wives are generally found to experience more burden than caregiving husbands, levels of distress among wives may diminish over time and approach levels of distress felt by husband caregivers (Zarit et al. 1986). Similarly, caregiving sons have been commonly found to experience less burden than do caregiving daughters (Horowitz 1985), and the latter are about three times more likely to become a caregiver (Coward and Dwyer 1990). Cross-generational studies have been more difficult to interpret. Some studies report few differences in burden between caregiving wives and daughters, whereas others report significant differences, especially in certain dimensions of burden (Cantor 1983; George and Gwyther 1986; Lawton et al. 1991; Price and Levy 1990; Quayhagen and Quayhagen 1988). Thus, for example, wives have been reported to manifest higher rates of psychological distress and personal burden, whereas daughters exhibit more role strain and interpersonal burden (Boutselis 1985). Finally, several studies have shown that black caregivers have lower levels of burden than white caregivers (Hinrichsen and Ramirez 1992; Lawton et al. 1992; Morycz et al. 1987; Mui 1992; Wood and Parham 1990). In most studies, however, controlling for socioeconomic factors led to the disappearance of differences.

Research on Effects of Behavior on Caregiver Distress

Partly because of the conceptual and methodological differences outlined above, there has been a lack of consistency in the literature with respect to the relationship between patients' behavior and caregiver distress. Most articles tended to find significant correlations between behavior and caregiver distress, usually in the moderate range of .20—.50 (e.g., George and Gwyther 1986; Hamel et al. 1990; Morycz 1985; Wilder et al. 1983; Zarit et al.

1986). Wilder and colleagues (1983) argue that "it is not dementia per se which is the important factor explaining family inconvenience, but rather the *behavior* [italics added] displayed that limits a family's activity" (p. 248).

On the other hand, some investigators are increasingly finding weak and nonsignificant correlates between behavior and caregiver distress (George and Gwyther 1986; Malonebeach and Zarit 1991; Miller and Montgomery 1990; Motenko 1989; Zarit et al. 1986), and they have underscored the caregiver's reactivity to symptomatology as a crucial intervening element: "Caregivers react differently to problem behaviors and vary in their skills for managing these problems. Further, all caregivers do not find the same problems to be troublesome" (Zarit et al. 1986, p. 265).

Different behaviors are also likely to elicit different levels of response among caregivers in general. For example, Quayhagen and Quayhagen (1988) found that only 8 of 29 behaviors generated moderate or severe stress for at least two-fifths of the caregivers surveyed. In order of frequency, they were as follows: repetitive questions, difficulty handling money, embarrassing things (primarily sexual), difficulty bathing, difficulty staying alone, difficulty cooking, dangerous behavior, and incontinence. Teri and colleagues (1992) observed that the most frequent patient behaviors did not necessarily elicit the strongest stressful reactions from caregivers. For example, "arguing" was seven times more common than "threats to hurt others," but the latter elicited much stronger reactions from caregivers. Similarly, appearing "anxious" was more commonly reported among patients than "comments about hopelessness"; the latter, however, elicited considerably stronger caregiver reactions. Reactions to behaviors also appear to vary among types of caregivers. Thus, the Quayhagens (1988) found that two of the behaviors described above—difficulty bathing and difficulty staying alone—caused daughters more stress, whereas "embarrassing things" caused wives more stress.

A handful of studies examined the effects of specific behaviors on caregiver distress. Such studies have been limited primarily to spousal caregivers. Wright (1991), for example, compared the marital quality of spouse pairs with an Alzheimer-afflicted partner with well-spouse control subjects. In this study, patients were in the early stages of dementia. Wright studied specific problem areas as well as patterns of coping. Management of finances was one such area; 31% of caregiver spouses reported the problem. Interestingly, similar problems were reported by well-spouse couples at an even higher rate (59%). This finding emphasizes that it is necessary to compare caregivers to non-caregivers if we want to determine whether caregiver problems are specific to the caregiver burden and not a concomitant of the normal aging process.

Spouses resorted to a range of coping responses. A few of the partners with Alzheimer's disease attempted to instruct their spouses to take over the financial responsibilities. Spouses without Alzheimer's disease handled the emotional reaction to their partners' loss of capability by having them continue to participate, but in a structured way; for example, the well spouses took over the management of the finances but had the spouses with Alzheimer's disease sign the checks. Problems were worse if the assumption of financial responsibility involved a role change for a spouse.

A majority of spousal caregivers experienced difficulties with sexual problems (Quayhagen and Quayhagen 1988). Among couples who were still sexually active, the mean frequency per month of sexual intimacy for couples older than 60 was 7.2 for the Alzheimer's disease group, whereas it was 2.4 for the well group (Wright 1991); the highest rates of sexual activity (14 or more times per month) were found in couples with a male spouse who had Alzheimer's disease.

There was significant variation in sexual initiation rates, and coping responses were related to them. When rates were low, spouses adapted by citing norms of aging. When moderate, half the couples were concordant on their satisfaction, but half complained of too much (childlike) affection or lack thereof. When sexual activity was high and was accompanied by clinging, demanding behavior (which occurred only in male spouses with Alzheimer's disease), wives generally expressed feeling exploited by their husbands and resentful toward them. This problem was compounded by the tendency of spouses with Alzheimer's disease to deny the problem and to be insensitive to their mates' feelings. Some wives also had to contend with the problem of leaving a sexually preoccupied husband at home when they wanted to take advantage of respite care, because the caregiver was almost invariably a female worker.

Yet another source of marital stress was spouses' repetitive questions and restless walking (Wright 1991). This produced tension and aggravation that caregivers tried to modulate through intense self-control, on the one hand, and displacement, on the other. Some spouses resorted to screaming into a pillow or locking themselves in the bathroom for privacy or prayer. Other spouses used limit setting, diversion, and taking respite time for themselves. When coping was unsuccessful, caregivers occasionally lost control and released their tension by screaming at the spouse, which tended to lead to feelings of guilt.

A Theoretical Model

How does patient behavior influence caregiver distress and institutionalization? Figure 12–1 provides a hypothetical path model of these relationships, based on the work of Wilder et al. (1983) and Pearlin et al. (1989, 1990). The model suggests that distress is

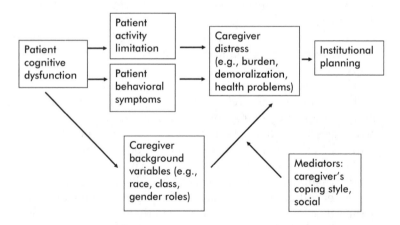

Figure 12–1. Theoretical model of the role of behavioral disturbance in caregiver distress.

the prime force in institutionalization and that the other variables act through distress. Moreover, the model proposes that among patient variables, cognitive dysfunction has little direct effect on distress; rather, it is behavioral symptoms and activity limitations that engender distress. Finally, the model incorporates the growing body of data showing that two mediators, coping functions and social networks, play an important role in moderating effects of various stressors, including behavioral problems.

Pearlin et al. (1989) have identified four coping functions: 1) prevention of the stressful situation—that is, the methods employed by the caregiver to avoid stressors; 2) management of the situation—that is, efforts to reduce the demands of caregiving or make them easier to perform; 3) management of the meaning of the situation—that is, how the situation is perceived and understood by the caregiver; 4) management of stress symptoms—that is, activities or behaviors used by the caregiver to deal with stressors. The Quayhagens (1988) found that specific coping strategies used by at least two-fifths of caregivers included help seeking and problem solving (i.e., management of the situation), existential growth (i.e., management of the meaning of the situation), and blame and fantasy (i.e., management of stress). Contrary to expectation, there were few differences in coping strategies among caregiving husbands, wives, and daughters, although not all coping strategies were equally effective for each type of caregiver. For example, problem solving and help seeking were associated with increased well-being among spouses but not among daughters. Further research is necessary to clarify these differing responses.

Although a theoretical role for social networks as a modifier of caregiver distress has frequently been proposed (Cohler et al. 1989; Pearlin et al. 1989; Zarit 1989), empirical support has been less definitive. On the positive side, Colerick and George (1986) and Morycz (1985) found that certain caregiver network variables diminished the likelihood of Alzheimer's disease patients' being institutionalized. Similarly, some researchers reported correlations between various social network measures and caregiver burden (Haley et al. 1987; Vitaliano et al. 1989; Zarit et al. 1980). Other investigators, however (Gilhooly 1984; Pruchno 1990; Teresi et al. 1988–1989; Zarit et al. 1986), have found no evidence that network variables affect caregivers' mental health or level of burden. Regrettably, much of this research has been limited to rudimentary network measures, and future studies must include more complex network dimensions (Cohen et al. 1990).

Intervention Techniques

Although the literature remains divided on the precise role behavioral problems play in caregiver distress, several surveys of caregivers have highlighted the importance caregivers assign to behavioral disturbances. For example, Smith and colleagues (1991) found that emotional and behavioral problems was one of the largest groups of pressing problems cited by caregivers. Similarly, Fortinsky and Hathaway (1990) found that behavioral management techniques were cited by three-fourths of caregivers as information that they considered extremely important. Hence, interventions to help caregivers deal with the effects of patients' behavior have become a critical part of the treatment armamentarium.

Although there are some differences between individual counseling and support groups for caregivers, their principal themes and objectives overlap considerably. Consonant with the theoretical model outlined above, both individual and group treatment can be seen as 1) acting directly on caregivers' distress by providing a setting to express emotional needs and feelings of guilt and inadequacy and 2) acting on intervening variables, such as coping and social networks, that have been found to buffer the effects of stressors such as behavior on the caregiver's level of distress.

It is possible to distill four principal themes typically addressed in individual counseling or support groups for caregivers (Smith et al. 1991; Toseland and Rossiter 1989):

1. Information
   - Information about the illness
   - Techniques for dealing with management problems
   - Techniques for dealing with patient physical safety and well-being

- Techniques for coping better with difficult activities of daily living, such as bathing and transferring
- Methods for obtaining additional personal assistance, entitlements, and respite services (e.g., day care, home care)

2. Emotional needs and self-care
   - Encouragement of better coping strategies for dealing with stresses of caregiving
   - Improvement in ability to deal with feelings of guilt, loneliness, inadequacy, and anger
   - Assistance in confronting conflicting emotions regarding institutionalization
   - Assistance in improving self-esteem; enabling caregivers to do more pleasurable things for themselves

3. Improvement of interpersonal relations and communications
   - Assistance in reducing interpersonal conflicts and relating better with the care receiver and other family members
   - Assistance in improving ability to cope with conflicting family roles and responsibilities

4. Development of support system
   - Helping caregivers learn about and feel comfortable with obtaining formal assistance and support from relatives
   - Encouraging caregivers to expand social activities and broaden social networks
   - Helping caregivers learn to use group members and the therapist as integral components of their network systems

Our clinical experience at the Brooklyn Alzheimer's Disease Assistance Center indicates that it is best to employ a multidisciplinary, multimodal approach to the management of caregiver distress. Our center's program addresses the educational and emotional aspects of distress through a six-pronged approach:

1. *Information and case management.* At the time of the initial assessment, caregivers are provided with oral, written, and audiotaped information about Alzheimer's disease support services (e.g., respite care, home aides), and entitlements. A

member of the social work staff is designated as the primary contact person and case manager. This worker helps coordinate needed resources and link the caregiver to them. Much of the initial effort is aimed at teaching caregivers about the stages of the disorder and the behaviors that commonly accompany each stage. We emphasize that these behaviors are generally not intentional but reflect underlying brain dysfunction. However, we also note that various interpersonal and environmental factors—such as caregiver hostility, overstimulation of patients, and new settings—can exacerbate or precipitate behavioral disturbance. Next, caregivers are also taught to define and circumscribe carefully the troubling behaviors so that specific strategies can be employed. Once problems are no longer viewed as global, but rather as specific and manageable, caregivers' distress usually dissipates.

2. *Support groups.* Caregivers are encouraged to attend a weekly support group in which members discuss techniques for handling behavioral problems and emotional concerns of the Alzheimer's disease patient.

3. *Activity groups.* Caregivers are encouraged to attend a weekly patient activity group to observe and learn techniques and activities for managing behavioral problems.

4. *Accessibility to professional assistance.* Caregivers are encouraged to call or meet frequently with social work staff and psychiatrists, who can assist with their concerns about the patient's behavior and illness as well as their own distress.

5. *Respite services.* Caregivers are encouraged to obtain in-home support services and to send the patient to a day program. Case managers work closely with the caregiver to link them with these services.

6. *Intensive individual, group, or family therapy.* For caregivers who are experiencing more persistent and serious emotional difficulties, referrals are made for individual or group psychotherapy or family therapy.

Well-controlled studies of counseling and support groups have appeared only within the past few years. These studies have yielded a mixed picture of the findings with respect to efficacy:

some studies reported no difference among wait-list, support, and family counseling groups (Haley 1991). Early case studies of single support groups reported success in glowing terms. However, a recent metanalytic review of the caregiver literature, using only controlled studies (Knight et al. 1993), indicated that group interventions had smaller effects than did individual interventions. Individual interventions had effects in the moderate range for both relief of caregiver burden and dysphoria; group interventions had effects in the low range.

One reason for the mixed success of support groups is the diversity of their approaches. Certain types of groups, such as those that are factual or information oriented, produce less satisfaction because they do not adequately meet the emotional needs of caregivers; nevertheless, informational groups are apparently very common. Future research needs to study support groups more systematically and take into account the group type. In addition, other variables need to be considered, such as the stage of the disease in the patients, the composition of the group in terms of age and gender, and the socioeconomic status of support recipients (Knight et al. 1993).

Ferris and co-workers (1987) demonstrated how an eight-point program of counseling for 41 families could be effective in influencing placement of a spouse or parent in a nursing home. Included in the counseling, which covered a 6-month period, was advice and assistance in getting auxiliary help, support groups, hooking the family up with community resources, and direct counseling and interventions with family members. The program resulted in consistent and marked reductions in emotional complaints—particularly depression, anger, anxiety, and insomnia—and consistent reduction in the incidence of physical complaints. Only one of the 41 families that initially had seriously considered nursing home placement actually placed their family member in a home. Such a program, targeting a specific group for specific intervention, appears to have been effective.

The impact of respite care (e.g., day care, in-home services, short inpatient stay) has been clouded by the fact that many studies have not been well controlled or may have included comparison groups receiving different types of respite services. However, when analysis was limited to studies with legitimate control groups, Knight and colleagues (1993) found a moderate effect for respite care in relieving caregiver burden and dysphoria. This finding is even more impressive because many of the respite programs reviewed were providing about 25%–50% of the effective amount of respite recommended by the Family Survival Project in California (Knight et al. 1993). This project had concluded that 8 hours per week was the minimum amount of respite required for achieving relief from caregiving workload.

Knight and co-workers have argued that a theoretical model is needed to guide interventions. It is not clear, for example, which type of intervention is likely to benefit a particular caregiver or how much intervention is necessary for achieving a desired effect. They conclude that "the past approach of throwing 'everything but the kitchen sink' into an intervention and evaluating this mixed approach at a minimal level of application is not helpful for the progress of science, practice, or policy" (p. 247).

Caregiving in the Broader Social Context

Most of the research in this area deals with caregiver burden at the level of individual families. It is also necessary to understand caregiving within a broader social context and to recognize the policy implications of some of the findings. Family caregiving has been viewed as a private good rather than as a social good (England et al. 1991). Public policy, therefore, has been to avoid extending benefits that would substitute government funds for home care that is currently provided "free" by friends and relatives. This policy ignores the facts that caregivers have no legal obligation to provide such care and that their ongoing consent to provide it saves society billions of dollars annually.

A decision to care for an impaired relative is made at enormous economic and psychological cost to caregivers. The responsibility of providing in-home personal and health-related tasks results in losses in other important areas of life, which presumably will have a lasting impact on them, their families, and society (England et al. 1991). Moreover, the fact that caregivers are predominantly women—72% of 2.3 million persons providing unpaid care are wives or adult daughters (Stone 1985)—impels us to consider the relationship between community care policies and gender justice. The 1982 National Long-Term Care Study reported that more than one-fifth of female caregivers had taken time off from work without pay to provide care (Stone et al. 1986), and another study found that 28% of the women who were staying home to care for their parent had quit work (Brody 1985). A study among corporate employees caring for elderly relatives found that women spent 16 hours weekly providing direct care, as contrasted with 5 hours for men (Ball and Greenberg 1985).

The current policy that provides public home care assistance only if it prevents institutionalization ignores the varying gradations of impairment. It also places caregivers in the unfortunate role of deciding between staying home to provide care and having their relative institutionalized.

Resistance to reforming community care policies has been based on three myths: 1) that people will cease or reduce their own caregiving efforts and let government take over; 2) that new programs will bring large new applicants out of the woodwork; 3) that family care saves the government money because it does not cost anything. Preliminary research has not substantiated these assumptions (Kane and Kane 1985; England et al. 1991; Weissert 1986). As England and associates (1991) recognize, "Without acknowledgment that family-provided care is a 'social good'—a contribution to society by women and men who often incur substantial personal, economic, and social costs—benefits for carers will continue to be minimal" (p. 240).

Summary

Despite a burgeoning of literature on caregiving in recent years, the specific effects of patient behavior on caregivers is relatively poorly understood. Considerable research will be needed before our understanding is complete. Among the more pressing issues to be considered are the following:

- The assessment of the impact of patients' behaviors on caregivers has been hindered by the lack of uniformity in 1) concepts of patient behavior and caregiver impact and 2) the variation in sample selection; for example, caregivers' age, gender, relationship, class, and ethnicity have all been found to affect level of impact.

- The correlation of patients' behavior with caregivers' distress has been in the moderate range, although some investigators have found low or no correlations. Many theorists now believe that it is necessary to examine more systematically the effects of coping and social network variables on caregiver distress.

- Individual and group programs to modify caregiver distress have focused on four themes: the provision of information, meeting emotional needs and self-care, improving interpersonal relations and communications, and developing support systems. Cumulatively, the evaluation of interventions for caregiver distress suggests that individual psychosocial and respite programs are moderately effective, group psychosocial programs less so. Studies have been limited by the diversity of their orientation and their subjects and by the absence of a guiding theoretical model.

- The impact of the broader social context on caregiving has been largely ignored and poorly studied. Family caregiving has been viewed as a private good rather than as a social good.

We have found that the most common reasons for caregivers to seek therapy are overwhelming symptoms of depression, anxiety, and anger that interfere with daily functioning or with their relationship with the patient. Typically, these symptoms may arise as part of the bereavement process surrounding the patient's illness; as a consequence of inadequate support from family, friends, or formal services; or as a product of a caregiver's lifelong coping styles. In most instances, symptoms can be relieved by short-term treatment. However, in a majority of cases, the stresses of caregiving may uncover deep-seated or characterological issues that require long-term treatment.

References

Alessi CA: Managing the behavioral problems of dementia in the home. Clin Geriatr Med 7:787–801, 1991

Ball GT, Greenberg B: The Travelers employee caregiver survey. Hartford, CT, The Travelers Company, Personnel Administration Department, 1985

Barusch AS, Spaid WM: Gender differences in caregiving: why do wives report greater burden? Gerontologist 29:667–675, 1989

Borden W, Berlin S: Gender coping and psychological well-being in spouses of older adults with chronic dementia. Am J Orthopsychiatry 60:603–610, 1990

Brody EM: Parent care as a normative family stress. Gerontologist 25:19–29, 1985

Brown LJ, Potter JF, Foster BG: Caregiver burden should be evaluated during geriatric assessment. J Am Geriatr Soc 38:455–460, 1990

Cantor MH: Strain among caregivers: a study of experience in the United States. Gerontologist 23:597–604, 1983

Cohen CI, Teresi J, Rosen S, et al: Alzheimer's disease and network reorganization. Paper presented at the annual scientific meeting of the Gerontological Society of America, Boston, MA, November 1990

Cohen-Mansfield J, Marx MS, Rosenthal AS: A description of agitation in a nursing home. J Gerontol 44:M77–M86, 1989

Cohen-Mansfield J, Billig N, Lipson S, et al: Medical correlates of agitation in nursing home residents. Gerontology 36:150–160, 1990

Cohler BJ, Groves L, Borden W, et al: Caring for family members with Alzheimer's disease, in Alzheimer's Disease Treatment and Family Stress: Directions for Research. Edited by Light E, Lebowitz B. Washington, DC, U.S. Government Printing Office, 1989, pp 50–105

Colerick EJ, George LK: Predictors of institutionalization among caregivers of patients with Alzheimer's disease. J Am Geriatr Soc 34:493–498, 1986

Coward RT, Dwyer JW: The association of gender, sibling network composition, and patterns of parent care by adult children. Research on Aging 12:158–181, 1990

Dura JR, Stukenberg KW, Kiecolt-Glaser JK: Anxiety and depressive disorders in adult children caring for demented parents. Psychol Aging 6:467–473, 1991

England SE, Keigher SM, Miller B, et al: Community care policies and gender justice, in Critical Perspectives on Aging: The Political and Moral Economy of Growing Old. Edited by Minkler M, Estes CL. Amityville, NY, Baywood, 1991, pp 227–244

Ferris SH, Steinberg G, Shulman E, et al: Institutionalization of Alzheimer's disease patients: reducing precipitating factors through family counseling. Home Health Care Services Quarterly 8:23–51, 1987

Fitting M, Rabins P, Lucas JL, et al: Caregivers for dementia patients: a comparison of husbands and wives. Gerontologist 26:248–252, 1986

Fortinsky RH, Hathaway TS: Information and service needs among active and former family caregivers of persons with Alzheimer's disease. Gerontologist 30:604–609, 1990

George LK, Gwyther LP: The dynamics of caregiver burden: changes in caregiver well-being over time. Paper presented at the annual scientific meeting of the Gerontological Society of America, San Antonio, TX, November 1984

George LK, Gwyther LP: Caregiver well-being: a multidimensional examination of family caregivers of demented adults. Gerontologist 26:253–259, 1986

Gilhooly MLM: The impact of care-giving on caregivers: factors associated with the psychological well-being of people supporting a dementing relative in the community. Br J Med Psychol 57:35–44, 1984

Haley WE: Caregiver intervention programs: the moral equivalent of free haircuts? Gerontologist 31:7–8, 1991

Haley WE, Pardo KM: Relationship of severity of dementia to caregiving stressors. Psychol Aging 4:389–392, 1989

Haley WE, Levine EG, Brown SL, et al: Stress, appraisal, coping, and social support as predictors of adaptational outcome among dementia caregivers. Psychol Aging 2:332–340, 1987

Hamel M, Gold DP, Andres D, et al: Predictors and consequences of aggressive behavior by community-based dementia patients. Gerontologist 30:206–211, 1990

Hinrichsen GA, Ramirez M: Black and white dementia caregivers: a comparison of their adaptation, adjustment, and service utilization. Gerontologist 32:375–381, 1992

Horowitz A: Sons and daughters as caregivers to older parents: differences in role performance and consequences. Gerontologist 25:612–617, 1985

Kane RL, Kane RA: A Will and a Way: What the United States Can Learn From Canada About Caring for the Elderly. New York, Columbia University Press, 1985, pp 19–26

Kinney JM, Stephens MAP: Hassles and uplifts of giving care to a family member with dementia. Psychol Aging 4:402–408, 1989

Knight BG, Lutzky SM, Macofsky-Urban F: A meta-analytic review of interventions for caregiver distress: recommendations for future research. Gerontologist 33:240–248, 1993

Lawton MP: The varieties of wellbeing, in Emotion in Adult Development. Edited by Malatesta CZ, Izard CE. Beverly Hills, CA, Sage, 1984, pp 67–84

Lawton PM, Moss M, Kleban MH, et al: A two-factor model of caregiving appraisal and psychological well-being. J Gerontol 46:P181–P189, 1991

Lawton PM, Rajagopal D, Brody E, et al: The dynamics of caregiving for a demented elder among black and white families. J Gerontol 47:S156–S164, 1992

Malonebeach EE, Zarit SH: Current research issues in caregiving to the elderly. Int J Aging Hum Dev 32:103–114, 1991

Miller B, Cafasso L: Gender differences in caregiving: fact or artifact? Gerontologist 32:498–507, 1992

Miller B, Montgomery A: Family caregivers and limitations in social activities. Research on Aging 12:72–93, 1990

Montgomery RJV, Hatch LR: The feasibility of volunteers and families forming a partnership for caregiving, in Families and Long-Term Care. Edited by Brubaker TH. Beverly Hills, CA, Sage, 1986

Montgomery RJV, Gonyea JG, Hooyman NR: Caregiving and the experience of subjective burden. Family Relations 34:19–26, 1985

Morycz RK: Caregiving strain and the desire to institutionalize family members with Alzheimer's disease. Research on Aging 7:320–361, 1985

Morycz RK, Malloy J, Bozich M, et al: Racial differences in family burden: clinical implication for social work. Gerontological Social Work 10:133–154, 1987

Motenko AK: The frustrations, gratifications, and well-being of dementia caregivers. Gerontologist 29:166–172, 1989

Mui AC: Caregiver strain among black and white daughter caregivers: a role theory perspective. Gerontologist 32:203–212, 1992

Parks SH, Pilisuk M: Caregiver burden: gender and the psychological costs of caregiving. Am J Psychiatry 61:501–509, 1991

Pearlin LI, Turner H, Semple S: Coping and the mediation of caregiver stress, in Alzheimer's Disease Treatment and Family Stress: Directions for Research. Edited by Light E, Lebowitz E. Washington, DC, U.S. Government Printing Office, 1989, pp 198–217

Pearlin LI, Mullan JT, Semple SJ, et al: Caregiving and the stress process: an overview of concepts and their measures. Gerontologist 30:583–594, 1990

Pillemer K, Suitor JJ: Violence and violent feelings: What causes them among family caregivers? J Gerontol 47:S165–S172, 1992

Poulshock SW, Deimling GT: Families caring for elders in residence: issues in the measurement of burden. J Gerontol 39:230–239, 1984

Price HJ, Levy KA: Variables influencing burden in spousal and adult child primary caregivers of persons with Alzheimer's disease in the home setting. The American Journal of Alzheimer's Care and Related Disorders and Research 5:34–43, 1990

Pruchno RA: The effects of help patterns on the mental health of spouse caregivers. Research on Aging 12:57–71, 1990

Quayhagen MP, Quayhagen M: Alzheimer's stress: coping with the caregiving role. Gerontologist 28:391–396, 1988

Smith GC, Smith MF, Toseland R: Problems identified by family caregivers in counseling. Gerontologist 31:15–21, 1991

Stone R: The feminization of poverty and older women: an update. Paper presented at the 113th annual meeting of the American Public Health Association, Washington, DC, November 1985Paper presented at the 113th annual meeting of the American Public Health Association, Washington, DC, November 1985

Stone R, Cafferata GL, Sangel J: Caregivers of the elderly: a national profile. Paper presented at the annual meeting of the American Society on Aging, San Francisco, CA, March 1986

Teresi J, Toner J, Bennett R, et al: Caregiver burden and long-term care planning. Journal of Applied Social Sciences 13:192–213, 1988–1989

Teri L, Truax P, Logsdon R, et al: Assessment of behavioral problems in dementia: the Revised Memory and Behavior Problems checklist. Psychol Aging 7:622–631, 1992

Toseland RW, Rossiter CM: Group interventions to support family caregivers: a review and analysis. Gerontologist 29:438–448, 1989

Townsend AL: Nursing home care and family caregivers' stress, in Stress and Coping in Later Life Families. Edited by Stephens MAP, Crowther JH, Hobfoll SE, et al. Washington, DC, Hemisphere, 1990

Vitaliano PP, Maturo RD, Ochs H, et al: A model of burden in caregivers of DAT patients, in Alzheimer's Disease Treatment and Family Stress: Directions for Research. Edited by Light E, Lebowitz B. Washington, DC, U.S. Government Printing Office, 1989, pp 267–291

Weissert WG: Seven reasons why it is so difficult to make community care cost-effective. Health Serv Res 20:421–433, 1986

Whitlach CJ, Zarit SH, von Eye A: Efficacy of interventions with caregivers: a reanalysis. Gerontologist 31:9–14, 1991

Wilder DE, Teresi JA, Bennett RG: Family burden and dementia, in The Dementias. Edited by Mayeux RI, Rosen WG. New York, Raven, 1983, pp 239–251

Wood JB, Parham IA: Coping with perceived burden: ethnic and cultural issues in Alzheimer's family caregiving. Journal of Applied Gerontology 9:325–339, 1990

Wright LK: The impact of Alzheimer's disease on the marital relationship. Gerontologist 31:224–237, 1991

Zarit SH: Issues and directions in family intervention research, in Alzheimer's Disease Treatment and Family Stress: Directions for Research. Edited by Light E, Lebowitz B. Washington, DC, U.S. Government Printing Office, 1989, pp 458–486

Zarit SH, Reever K, Bach-Peterson J: Relatives of the impaired elderly: correlates of feelings of burden. Gerontologist 20:649–655, 1980

Zarit SH, Orr NK, Zarit JM: Working With Families of Dementia Victims: a Treatment Manual. Washington, DC, U.S. Department of Health and Human Services, Administration on Aging, 1983

Zarit SH, Todd PA, Zarit JM: Subjective burden of husbands and wives as caregivers: a longitudinal study. Gerontologist 26:260–266, 1986

CHAPTER 13

Long-Term Care and the Behaviorally Disturbed Patient

Lorna S. Carlin, M.D.
Brian A. Lawlor, M.D., F.R.C.P.I., M.R.C.Psych.

*I*t is often the behavioral disturbances complicating Alzheimer's disease that compel families and physicians to seek long-term care for Alzheimer's disease patients. Behaviors such as agitation and oppositional, combative responses toward caregivers can become impossible to deal with on a 24-hour basis. Relentless pacing, wandering, and searching for misplaced items slowly grind the caregiver down. Restless nights secondary to sleep disturbance in the Alzheimer's disease patient can often spur the caregiver to request respite and eventually seek long-term care. This tragic progression of disturbed behaviors associated with Alzheimer's disease imposes increasing stress on the primary caregiver, and although it may initially be contained within the family, inevitably the caregiver must enlist outside help. Very few families give up their loved ones easily, and generally only when the burden of care has gone beyond the breaking point.

Removing the patient from the community to an institutional setting may alleviate the burden for the caregiver, but the behavioral disturbance will continue to affect patient management in the nursing home. Because more than 75% of nursing home residents with dementia exhibit a behavioral complication (Cohen-

Mansfield 1986; Rovner et al. 1986), the management and containment of the behaviorally disturbed Alzheimer's disease patient in the long-term care setting is a matter of great import from a national and international point of view. This chapter focuses on the need of behaviorally disturbed Alzheimer's disease patients for long-term care in the community and nursing home, the response of long-term care facilities to the immense problems posed by behavioral disturbance, and the health care policy attention that these complex issues warrant.

Behavioral Complications in Alzheimer's Disease and the Need for Long-Term Care

Long-term care exists along a continuum that begins in the home with family and friends and can involve a large and varied spectrum of services, including home care, home help services, social and housing programs, ambulatory care, acute care, and nursing home care (Evaswick 1988). Unfortunately, long-term care has become almost synonymous with institutionalization because of the paucity and poor quality of community long-term care services.

Although Alzheimer's patients with particularly good family and community support systems may be able to remain home for years, Alzheimer's disease patients in the middle and late stages of the disease will often require home health services almost on a 24-hour basis. Even where extensive supports are in place, community care of Alzheimer's disease patients can break down for a myriad of reasons. Often the caregiver is a spouse who is also elderly and frail and has medical problems and so cannot coordinate care even with significant home help. The patient may be widowed or never married, having no remaining family network. Thus, even with supportive, involved family, behavioral symptoms become overwhelming as capacity is lost for the fundamental activities of daily living (ADL).

Currently, the principal constraints for a family who wants to maintain a patient at home are community resources that are inadequate to alleviate what becomes an unmanageable burden for the family. The Omnibus Budget Reconciliation Act (1981) allowed funds that had been restricted to nursing home care to be applied to community care. As long as the Medicaid budget remains constant, however, the nursing home is often the only, and actually the less expensive, option once intensive care is required (Kane and Kane 1990).

Behavioral Disturbance and the Need to Place Alzheimer's Disease Patients

The behavioral disturbances that most frequently necessitate placement and that cannot be managed in a community setting are daytime and nighttime wandering and incontinence. These behaviors are resistant to pharmacological or environmental intervention in the community and require intense personnel input, through either direct one-to-one supervision (e.g., for wandering) or continued basic nursing intervention (incontinence). Incontinence of bladder and bowel is an inevitable part of the progressive loss of autonomous functioning in Alzheimer's disease. This is the symptom that often triggers the decision for placement in a nursing home (Harris 1986). Other behaviors that become unmanageable in the community or family setting include violent or aggressive outbursts that threaten the safety of others and verbally disruptive behaviors such as persistent screaming.

Interestingly, all these problematic behaviors tend to be associated with more severe dementia and increased dependency needs. In general, violent and agitated patients tend to be more dependent (Deutsch et al. 1991) and have lower cognitive scores (Cooper et al. 1990). This is not simply an effect of cognitive impairment, however, and it may be that the co-occurrence of behavioral complications produces a greater degree of functional impairment and dependency.

Verbally loud and disruptive behavior often continues to be a problem in the nursing home setting. Screaming is done by at least 25% of nursing home residents (Deutsch et al. 1991), the majority of whom have Alzheimer's disease. These Alzheimer's disease patients tend to be the most severely affected, and they have the greatest need for help with basic ADL. It is actually when these patients are getting help with bathing and toileting that the screaming behavior is at its worst.

Institutional Care for Alzheimer's Disease Patients

With regard to the long-term placement of behaviorally disturbed Alzheimer's disease patients, the majority are in proprietary nursing homes. In the past there was a reluctance to admit Alzheimer's disease patients to nursing homes because of high dependency needs and management problems. This situation has been alleviated by the recent change in formulas for reimbursement, which are now more sensitive to costs in terms of staff time necessary to care for Alzheimer's disease patients with a multiplicity of ADL and behavioral problems.

A significant minority of Alzheimer's disease patients end up being cared for in state psychiatric hospitals. It appears that Alzheimer's disease patients, at a conservative estimate, constitute about 5% of all state hospital patients. They are usually transferred to these hospitals from nursing homes for control of unmanageable behavior. Once again, it is the behavioral complications of this illness that necessitate placement in state psychiatric facilities; the most common reasons given for referral are behaviors such as hitting, wandering, yelling, smearing and throwing (Moak and Fisher 1990). Civil commitment is another means of admission for incompetent patients to psychiatric hospitals from the community, because mental health law does not give the court jurisdiction over nursing homes, which are usually unlocked and voluntary.

Institutional Response to the Behaviorally Disturbed Alzheimer's Disease Patient

In the nursing home, behavioral symptoms frequently result in the employment of restraints to modify activity. This is a concern of caregivers working in long-term care facilities as well as of government. One internal study found that at a long-term care facility, residents with Alzheimer's disease were physically restrained between 8.5 and 14 hours a day while awake (Maas 1988). In addition, chemical restraints in the form of psychotropic medication are often employed for behavioral management. A survey in two dementia units in a Midwestern nursing home found that 62% of patients were taking psychotropic medication, with 43% taking neuroleptics, 17% prescribed antianxiety medication or sedative-hypnotics, and 7% antidepressants (Taft and Barken 1990). Concern about misuse of neuroleptics as chemical restraints has resulted in a federal response as part of the Omnibus Budget Reconciliation Act (1987) regulations. These regulatory guidelines went into effect in October 1990 and require a minimum of monthly audits by a licensed pharmacist. Noncompliance with guidelines must be reported to designated personnel, and violations may result in decertification by Medicaid. The goal is to reduce the use of chemical restraints and discontinue these medications whenever possible (Omnibus Budget Reconciliation Act 1987).

As caregiver strategies and modified environments to manage the behavioral symptoms of Alzheimer's disease develop, the reliance on restraints should diminish. Nursing homes have been instrumental in developing and managing special care units for patients with Alzheimer's disease. These units are modified to reduce wandering by eliminating long hallways. A wanderer's lounge can be provided to allow agitated patients an unrestrained but safe pacing area. Attention is given to minimizing confusing stimuli such as mirrors, bold patterns, and overhead speakers. There are no sharp edges, beds are closer to the floor to prevent injurious falls, and rooms are individualized with belongings from the patient's past. Staff are educated to attend to the special needs of these residents, and they are taught methods to cope with their own emotional response, reduce stress, and forestall burnout. Based on a national survey, it was estimated that 7.6% of nursing homes had special care units and as many as 14% planned to have them by 1991 (Leon et al. 1989). This growth is occurring along with studies to determine whether there is empirical support for the proliferation of special care units and whether it is advantageous to separate this population from the other residents in the nursing home (Sloane and Mathew 1991).

There have been no controlled studies examining the efficacy of these units, although there is some evidence that they can be helpful in decreasing combativeness (Rovner et al. 1990).

Financial Implications

The National Foundation for Brain Research (1992) recently reported that direct and indirect costs for dementia exceed the costs of cancer and coronary artery disease and that the costs of dealing with Alzheimer's disease equal those of the entire Medicare program. Long-term care provided by nursing homes figures largely in these expenses. A prospective study assessing nursing home and hospital use by Alzheimer's disease patients has demonstrated that the combination of the high rate of nursing home entry and lengthy stays makes long-term care the largest determinant of the cost of care in Alzheimer's disease (Welch et al. 1992): 75% of the cohort eventually resided in a nursing home during the study period, at an estimated cost per patient (during the study period) ranging from $39,000 to $56,000.

These frightening financial figures have led policymakers to the rationale of attempting to restrict the number of nursing home beds, in the belief that community care is a less costly and more desirable approach to long-term care. However, false logic may be operating here, as illustrated by a U.S. General Accounting Office (1983) study showing that the cost of community care for severely impaired elderly people is actually higher than the nursing home cost.

Furthermore, when nursing home beds are not available, costs to other parts of the health care system are increased. If a patient is ready for discharge from a hospital, but no nursing home bed is available, unnecessary hospital days accumulate. The Hospital Insurance Trust Fund spends more than a billion dollars a year in acute-care hospital fees for those waiting to enter a nursing home. Alzheimer's disease undoubtedly accounts for a significant proportion of that cost, because the longest-staying patients tend to be eligible for Medicaid, to have behavioral problems, and to be incontinent and disoriented. The problem is being exacerbated by limited nursing home sites. The current long-term care system is barely adequate to provide for the existing Alzheimer's disease patients and may fail markedly in the future if health care policy reforms are not forthcoming.

Recommendations and Conclusions

What are the implications for long-term care policy of behavioral complications in Alzheimer's disease? It would appear that there are varying thresholds that necessitate admission to a long-term care facility. Some of these factors are intrinsic to the disease in the individual patient, whereas some are extrinsic and refer more to the availability of community and family supports and to the durability of the caregiver. The provision of adequate community facilities to assess and manage behaviorally disturbed patients is necessary to reduce the considerable burden on caregivers and families. This might prevent the prolonged occupation of an acute-care bed by an Alzheimer's disease patient and allow the continued management of the patient in the community. However, it is also important to recognize that easier access by behaviorally disturbed Alzheimer's disease patients to nursing home beds could actually save money, because the point is reached when it no longer becomes feasible or cost effective to continue to maintain a patient in the community.

References

Cohen-Mansfield J: Agitated behaviors in the elderly, II: preliminary results in the cognitively deteriorated. J Am Geriatr Soc 34:722–727, 1986

Cooper JK, Mungas D, Weiler PG: Relation of cognitive status and abnormal behavior in AD. J Am Geriatr Soc 38:867–870, 1990

Deutsch LH, Bylsma F, Rovner BW et al: Psychosis and physical aggression in probable Alzheimer's disease. Am J Psychiatry 148:1159–1163, 1991

Evaswick C: The continuum of long term care, in Introduction to Health Series, 3rd Edition. Edited by Williams SJ, Torrens PR. New York, Wiley, 1988, pp 219–223

Harris T: Aging in the eighties: prevalence and impact of urinary problems in individuals age 65 years and over. NCHS Advanced Data 121:1–8, August 27, 1986

Kane RL, Kane RA: Health care for older people: organizational and policy issues, in Handbook of Aging and Social Sciences, 3rd Edition. Edited by Binstock RH, George LK. New York, Academic Press, 1990, pp 415–437

Leon J, Potter DEB, Cunningham PJ: Availability of special nursing home programs for Alzheimer's disease patients. Unpublished manuscript. National Center for Health Services Research and Health Care Technology Assessment, Rockville, MD, 1989

Maas M: Management of patients with Alzheimer's disease in long term care facilities. Nursing Clinics of North America 23:57–68, 1988

Moak GS, Fisher WH: Alzheimer's disease and related disorders in state mental hospitals: data from a nationwide survey. Gerontologist 30:798–802, 1990

National Foundation for Brain Research Report: The Cost of Disorders of the Brain. Washington, DC, National Foundation for Brain Research, 1992

Omnibus Budget Reconciliation Act (U.S. Public Law 97-35). Washington, DC, U.S. Government Printing Office, 1981

Omnibus Budget Reconciliation Act (U.S. Public Law 100-203). Washington, DC, U.S. Government Printing Office, 1987

Rovner BW, Kafonek S, Filipp L, et al: Prevalence of mental illness in a community nursing home. Am J Psychiatry 143:1446–1449, 1986

Rovner BW, Blaustein M, Folstein MF, et al: Stability over one year in patients admitted to a nursing home dementia unit. Int J Geriatr Psychiatry 15:77–82, 1990

Sloane PD, Mathew LJ (eds): Dementia Units in Long Term Care. Baltimore, MD, Johns Hopkins University Press, 1991, pp xiii–xx

Taft LB, Barken RL: Drug abuse? Use and misuse of psychotropic drugs in AD. Journal of Gerontological Nursing 16:4–10, 1990

U.S. General Accounting Office: Medicaid and Nursing Home Care: Cost Increases and the Need for Services Are Creating Problems for the States and the Elderly. Washington, DC, U.S. Government Printing Office, 1983

Welch HG, Walsh JS, Larson EB: The cost of institutional care in AD: nursing home and hospital use in a prospective cohort. J Am Geriatr Soc 40:221–224, 1992

Index

*Page numbers printed in **boldface** type refer to tables or figures.*